Dysphagia: Diagnosis and Management

Edited by
Michael E. Groher

BUTTERWORTHS
Boston • London
Sydney • Wellington • Durban • Toronto

Every effort has been made to ensure that the drug dosage schedules within this text are accurate and conform to standards accepted at time of publication. However, as treatment recommendations vary in the light of continuing research and clinical experience, the reader is advised to verify drug dosage schedules herein with information found on product information sheets. This is especially true in cases of new or infrequently used drugs.

Library of Congress Cataloging in Publication Data
Main entry under title:

Dysphagia: diagnosis and management.

  Includes index.
  1. Deglutition disorders—Handbooks, manuals, etc.
I. Groher, Michael E.   [DNLM: 1. Deglutition disorders—
Diagnosis—Handbooks.   2. Deglutition disorders—Therapy—
Handbooks. WI 39 D998]
RC815.2.D87 1984   617'.533   84–3211
ISBN 0–409–95112–9

Butterworth Publishers
80 Montvale Avenue
Stoneham, MA 02180

10 9 8 7 6 5 4

Printed in the United States of America

This book is dedicated to the memory of David P. Osborne, Jr., M.D., whose life was tragically ended while serving as the coeditor of this volume in its beginning stages. In many ways he was the inspiration for its completion. He taught me much about living, and for that I always will be grateful.

Michael E. Groher

CONTENTS

CONTRIBUTORS

Ina Elfant Asher, M.S., O.T.R.
Instructor, Thomas Jefferson
University, Department of
Occupational Therapy, College of
Allied Health Sciences,
Philadelphia, Pennsylvania

Jeffrey A. Buckwalter, M.D.
Chief Resident, Section of
Otolaryngology, Department of
Surgery, Yale University School
of Medicine, New Haven,
Connecticut

Abby S. Bloch, M.S., R.D.
Head, Clinical Nutrition Support
Kitchen, Memorial Sloan-
Kettering Cancer Center,
New York

Susan M. Fleming, Ph.D.
Director, Clinical Deglutition and
Research Section, Veterans
Administration Medical Center,
Allen Park, Michigan; Clinical
Appointee, Rehabilitation
Institute, and Departments of
Surgery, Harper Hospital and
Wayne State University, Detroit,
Michigan

Barbara A. Griggs, M.A., R.N.
Coordinator, Hyperalimentation
Unit, New York Hospital-Cornell
Medical Center, New York;
honorary member, Nursing Board
of Advisors for the American
Society for Parenteral and Enteral
Nutrition

Michael E. Groher, Ph.D.
Assistant Chief, Audiology and
Speech Pathology, Veterans
Administration Medical Center,
New York; Associate Clinical
Professor, New York University,
C. W. Post University, and
Adelphi University, New York

Robert M. Miller, Ph.D.
Staff member, Veterans
Administration Medical Center,
Seattle, Washington; Clinical
Assistant Professor, Departments
of Rehabilitation Medicine and
Speech and Hearing Sciences,
University of Washington, Seattle

Roger M. Morrell, M.D., Ph.D.
Chief, Neurology Service,
Veterans Administration Medical
Center, Allen Park, Michigan;
Professor of Neurology/
Immunology and Microbiology,
Wayne State University, Detroit,
Michigan; Kellogg Foundation
International Scholar (Alzheimer's
Disease) of the Institute of
Gerontology, University of
Michigan, Ann Arbor

Harold C. Pillsbury III, M.D.
Associate Professor and Chief,
Division of Otolaryngology,
Department of Surgery, University
of North Carolina at Chapel Hill

PREFACE

Health care providers agree that good nutrition is a prerequisite for maintaining and improving health and that receiving this nutrition orally is most expedient and psychologically pleasurable. It is surprising then that only in the past decade have we begun in earnest systematically to evaluate and treat patients with swallowing disorders in an effort to provide quality nutritional care. This book explores our most recent efforts.

Prior to the early 1970s, patients incapable of swallowing were managed by feeding gastrostomy or by nasogastric tube feedings. Return to oral feeding was a primary goal, but attempts to move in this direction were halfhearted, partly from ignorance, partly from lack of time. To complicate matters, no one person had direct responsibility for monitoring patients' feeding and swallowing.

Health care professionals have discovered in recent years, however, that active intervention with dysphagic patients, including carefully planned diagnostic evaluations and subsequent management and rehabilitative techniques, often assists a patient's return to normal feeding and swallowing; a result that speeds recovery and enhances the quality of life.

It is apparent to me that our efforts to provide this care require close cooperation of a professional, multidisciplinary staff, wherein each member possesses particular expertise. It is the combined expertise that links diagnosis and treatment. A diagnosis is established through cooperation between the physician with primary care responsibility and consultants in neurology, radiology, gastroenterology, surgery, and psychiatry. Further evaluation by the nurse and speech pathologist is critical to measure level of function and to follow the rate of improvement during treatment sessions. The dietitian and therapist must join forces to ensure adherence to dietary requirements and appropriateness of food formula and consistency. The speech pathologist, physical therapist, and occupational therapist must design and implement a program of rehabilitation tailored to each individual, always in cooperation with the nursing staff who are responsible for daily management of the patient.

Because dysphagia management involves multiple disciplines, our basic core of knowledge is dispersed among many different journals, making it difficult for the beginning clinician to read about and understand the current state of the art. As the clinicians and researchers at the Johns Hopkins Swallowing Center have remarked, "The feeding process . . . is located at the intersection of various medical disciplines, but it has not been adequately addressed by any of them."

Here we attempt to combine this knowledge, with emphasis on treatment. Contained in this volume is a representative sampling of approaches currently practiced by each member of the dysphagia rehabilitation team. We hope it will be a valuable resource in the diagnosis and treatment of swallowing disorders.

While knowledge in this field is still new and empirical data are lacking, I am confident that the current interest in dysphagia management will spur the necessary investigations to continue our efforts in establishing successful diagnostic and treatment protocols for these patients.

We do know that disorders of the swallowing mechanism can result from a broad spectrum of disabilities. These disorders range from minimal difficulty swallowing foods and liquids to inability to swallow without a high risk of aspiration in a patient who may require a gastrostoma or feeding tube for nutritional maintenance. At one extreme the disability is severe, the cause usually clear, and the therapy urgent. At the other are patients with mild to moderate dysphagia, no clear diagnosis, but a significant disability that may become life-threatening. This book is written with both groups of patients in mind.

While our focus is the adult population, clinicians working in the pediatric sector will benefit especially from chapters on diagnosis, evaluation, and program development. Some management and rehabilitative techniques do not directly apply to infants and children, but certain conceptual frameworks do—for example, the importance of diet modification.

Throughout the text, the distinction between neurologic and mechanical disorders of the swallowing mechanism is maintained. This is done for several reasons. Diagnostically, the two categories often are mutually exclusive, and attempts to classify the more subtle disorders should be made with this separation in mind. The distinction is also valid in therapy, since the techniques used for neurologic disorders differ from those used for mechanical disorders. From the outset, the careful clinician must have the differential diagnosis of dysphagia clearly in mind, and not stop after the first few common disorders have been ruled out. To leave a patient with no diagnosis or to conclude that the origin is psychiatric when persistent investigation would uncover a treatable cause is the pitfall that we hope this resource will help clinicians avoid.

It is my firm conviction that resorting immediately to tube or gastrostomy feedings in cases of dysphagia is a mistake, particularly if the condition has not been adequately diagnosed and other therapeutic measures have not been tried. The limitations and the compromise of quality of life that this presents to the patient are unacceptable.

Not all patients will respond to our rehabilitative efforts; however, improved management of their swallowing dysfunction short of total rehabilitation should not be underestimated. The importance of delivering adequate nutrition to hospitalized patients, particularly those who cannot receive nourishment by mouth, should be clear to all who invest their time with this patient group. More rapid wound healing, a briefer hospital stay, and an improved psychological outlook for the patient are important dividends.

Techniques used in establishing a clear diagnosis followed by the development of creative and realistic treatment protocols require in-depth didactic preparation and clinical exposure. They require a well-trained staff for implementation, cooperation on the part of the patient and family, considerable time and patience, and most important, a team approach.

Michael Groher
New York

PART I

Pathology and Evaluation of Swallowing Disorders

CHAPTER 1

The Neurology of Swallowing
Roger M. Morrell

This chapter gives a detailed description of the act of swallowing, including the fundamental anatomic requirements for normal swallowing, especially arrangements of bones and muscles comprising the oropharynx. In addition, the neural mechanisms and anatomy as well as the neuromuscular control mechanisms involved in swallowing are described. A brief introduction is given to physiologic aspects related to the act of swallowing, such as changes in pressure in various segments of the buccal cavity, oropharynx, and esophagus. The chapter does not cover details of the regulation of hunger and appetite.

THE NORMAL SWALLOW

Normal swallowing involves three separate stages: (1) voluntary transfer of material from the mouth to the pharynx; (2) involuntary (reflex-dependent), highly coordinated transport of material away from the mouth or buccal cavity by a contraction wave of the pharyngeal constrictor muscles, past a relaxed cricopharyngeus muscle into the upper esophagus; and (3) the transport (also involuntary) of material along the esophagus through a relaxed lower esophageal sphincter into the gastric cardia (Figure 1.1). It is important to remember that the anatomic arrangement mediating swallowing involves the pharyngeal tract, a cavity common to both respiration and deglutition. The anatomic and physiologic aspects of this highly complex and virtually unconscious act deserve particular attention.

The oral cavity extends from the lips anteriorly to the pharynx posteriorly and contains the tongue, gums, and teeth. It is separated from the nasal cavity by the hard palate and muscular soft palate. The muscular pharynx communicates between and joins the nasal and oral cavities. The nasopharynx lies above the soft palate and the oropharynx lies posterior to the mouth. The pharynx extends below to the esophagus; its inferior portion is called the hypopharynx or laryngopharynx and is separated from the esophagus by the cricopharyngeus muscle. The cartilaginous larynx lies anterior to the hypopharynx at the upper end of the trachea, suspended by

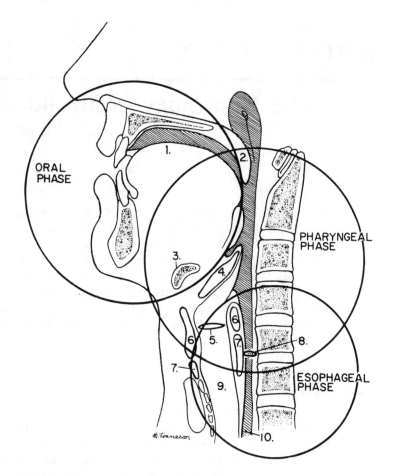

Figure 1.1. The normal swallow involves three separate
stages that are interdependent and highly coordinated:
(1) tongue, (2) soft palate, (3) hyoid bone, (4) epiglottis,
(5) vocal folds, (6) thyroid cartilage, (7) cricoid cartilage,
(8) pharyngoesophageal sphincter, (9) trachea, and
(10) esophagus. Reprinted by permission of the publisher and
the author, from Schultz et al., 1979.

muscles attached to the hyoid bone. The cricoid cartilage lies above the
trachea with the thyroid cartilage above it. Both are suspended from muscles
attached to the hyoid. Internally, the larynx contains the epiglottis projecting
into the pharyngeal cavity. Between it and the base of the tongue is a recess
called the vallecula (Figure 1.2). The vocal and vestibular folds are also
contained within the larynx. The vocal folds are below the bulkier vestibular
folds. Their anterior attachment is at the thyroid cartilage. Posteriorly, they

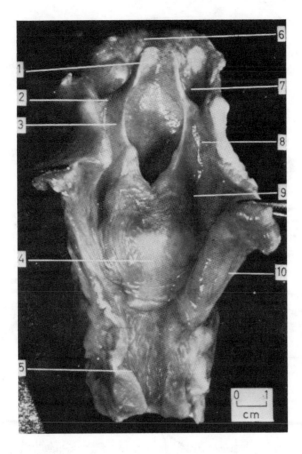

Figure 1.2.   The vallecular (7) and pyriform spaces (8, 9) are potential sites for abnormal retention of food and liquid. Note their relationship to other laryngeal structures: (1) epiglottis; (2) pharyngo-epiglottic fold; (3) aryepiglottic fold; (4) postcricoid region; (5) cervical esophagus; (6) base of tongue; (10) posterolateral pharyngeal wall. Reprinted by permission of the publisher, from Ballantyne and Groves, 1971.

attach to the vocal process of the arytenoid cartilages. The pyriform sinuses are recesses between the larynx and the hypopharyngeal wall (see Figure 1.2).

Neuromuscular Actions

Neuromuscular actions described in the following section depend on the bony and muscular structure of the head and neck (Figure 1.3). As stated

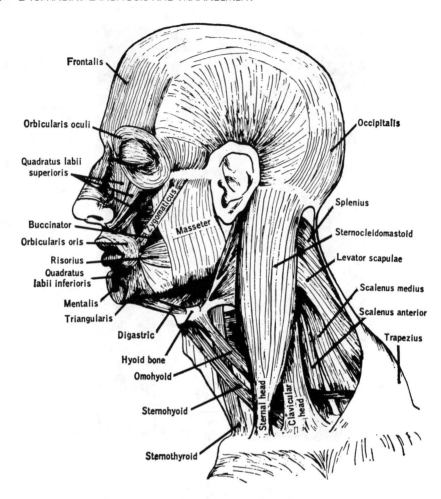

Figure 1.3. Relationships between the bony and muscular structures active in the normal swallow. Reprinted by permission of the publisher, from Kaplan, Anatomy and physiology of speech, McGraw-Hill Book Company, © 1960.

previously, the horseshoe-shaped hyoid bone supports the tongue and larynx. Above it lies the mandible or lower jaw that is highly mobile, consisting of a U-shaped body containing important ridges for muscle attachments. The upper jaw or maxilla is adjacent to the floor of the orbit of the eye. It meets the zygomatic or cheek bone and is adjoined by the L-shaped palatine bones lying posterior to the nasal cavity. The perpendicular part of the palatines forms the back of the nasal cavity while the horizontal part forms the back of the hard palate (the bony roof of the mouth). Important muscles of the face, neck, tongue, and pharynx attach to the temporal bone, which has five major portions. Major muscle attachments of importance are also related to the pterygoid processes of the sphenoid bone, which project inferiorly and support the internal or medial and external or lateral pterygoid muscles. Together with the masseter and temporalis muscles, pterygoid muscles are the primary muscles of chewing and are innervated by the mandibular branch of the trigeminal nerve (Table 1.1). The masseter closes the jaw while the temporalis moves it up, forward, or backward. The internal pterygoid muscles work bilaterally to elevate the mandible while unilaterally they shift the jaw to the opposite side. The external pterygoid muscles work together, pulling down or forward while unilaterally moving the jaw or chin to the opposite side. Both sets of pterygoid muscles cooperate to grind in mastication. The major facial muscles (Table 1.2), especially the buccinator, compress the lips and flatten the cheeks in the movement of food across the teeth. They are innervated by the facial nerve. The buccinator fibers blend with those of the orbicularis oris—the sphincter of the lips.

Proceeding inferiorly, the suprahyoid group of muscles (Table 1.3) consists of the geniohyoid, which draws the hyoid bone up and forward depressing the jaw; and the mylohyoid, which elevates the hyoid bone and tongue and depresses the jaw. These are innervated by the hypoglossal and trigeminal nerves respectively. The digastric muscles contain an anterior and a posterior belly. The anterior belly is innervated by the mandibular branch

Table 1.1. Muscles of Mastication.

Muscle	Origin	Insertion	Nerve	Action
Temporalis	Temporal fossa of skull	Ramus and co-ronoid pro-cess of mandible	Trigeminal	Elevates or closes mandi-ble, retracts mandible
Masseter	Zygomatic arch	Ramus of man-dible	Trigeminal	Elevates or closes mandi-ble
Medial	Palatine bone, lateral ptery-goid plate, tuberosity of maxilla	Ramus of man-dible	Trigeminal	Elevates or closes mandi-ble
Lateral ptery-goid	Great wing of sphenoid and lateral ptery-goid plate	Neck of con-dyle of man-dible	Trigeminal	Depressor or opener of mandible, protrudes mandible, permits side-to-side movement of mandible

Table 1.2.   Muscles of the Face.

Muscle	Origin	Insertion	Nerve	Action
Orbicularis oris	Neighboring muscles, mostly buccinator; has many layers of tissue around the lips	Skin around lips and angles of the mouth	Facial	Closes, opens, protrudes, inverts, and twists lips
Zygomaticus minor	Zygomatic bone	Orbicularis oris in upper lip	Facial	Draws upper lip upward and outward
Levator labii superioris	Below infraorbital foramen in maxilla	Orbicularis oris in upper lip	Facial	Pulls up or elevates upper lip
Levator labii superioris alaeque nasi	Process of maxilla	Skin at mouth angle, orbicularis oris	Facial	Raises angle of the mouth
Zygomaticus major	Zygomatic bone	Fibers of the orbicularis oris, angle of the mouth	Facial	Draws upper lip upward, draws angle of mouth upward and backward; the smiling muscle
Levator anguli oris (caninus)	Canine fossa of maxilla	Lower lip near angle of the mouth	Facial	Pulls down corners of mouth
Depressor anguli oris	Outer surface and above lower border of mandible	Skin of cheek, corner of mouth, lower border of mandible	Facial	Draws lower lip down, draws angle of mouth down and inward
Depressor labii inferioris	Lower border of the mandible	Skin of lower lip, orbicularis oris	Facial	Depresses lower lip
Mentalis	Incisor fossa of mandible	Skin of chin	Facial	Pushes up lower lip, raises chin
Risorius	Platysma, fascia over the masseter skin	Angle of mouth, orbicularis oris	Facial	Draws corners or angle of mouth outward, causes dimples,

Table 1.2.   *(continued)*

Muscle	Origin	Insertion	Nerve	Action
Risorius (cont.)				gives expression of strain to face
Buccinator	Alveolar process of maxilla, buccinator ridge of mandible	Angle of mouth, orbicularis oris	Facial	Flattens cheek, holds food in contact with teeth, retracts angles of the mouth

of the trigeminal nerve and depresses the jaw or raises the hyoid, whereas the posterior portion is innervated by the facial nerve and elevates or retracts the hyoid. The stylohyoid muscle elevates the hyoid during swallowing; the hyoglossus and the genioglossus, as laryngeal elevators and extrinsic tongue muscles, depress the tongue or help to elevate the hyoid bone when the tongue is fixed. Both are innervated by the hypoglossal nerve. The styloglossus draws the tongue up and back during swallowing while the palatoglossus raises the back of the tongue and lowers the sides of the soft palate. These are innervated by the hypoglossal and accessory nerves respectively. The tongue itself contains four separate muscle masses that have different effects on the shape, contour, and function of the tongue. All are innervated by the hypoglossal nerve.

Five muscles related to the soft palate adjust its position (Table 1.4). These are the palatoglossal; levator veli palatini (pharyngeal plexus and accessory nerve), which elevates the soft palate and seals the nasopharynx; and the tensor veli palatini (mandibular branch of the trigeminal nerve), which tenses the palate and dilates the orifice of the auditory tube. The palatopharyngeus muscle (pharyngeal plexus and spinal accessory nerve) depresses the soft palate, approximates the palate or pharyngeal folds, and constricts the pharynx. The muscularis uvula (spinal accessory nerve) shortens the soft palate.

At the rear of the throat is the muscular pharynx (Figure 1.4) whose superior, middle, and inferior constrictor muscles constitute its external circular layer and work together to "strip" a bolus of food toward the esophagus during swallowing. Each constrictor is innervated by the vagus and spinal accessory nerves. Three other muscles constitute the internal longitudinal layer of the pharynx: the palatopharyngeus, stylopharyngeus, and salpingopharyngeus. The stylopharyngeus (glossopharyngeal nerve) elevates the pharynx and to some extent the larynx during swallowing, while the salpingopharyngeus (accessory nerve and pharyngeal plexus) draws the lateral walls of the pharynx up (Table 1.5).

Table 1.3.   Suprahyoid Muscles.

Muscle	Origin	Insertion	Nerve	Action
Mylohyoid (anterior belly digastric)	Inner surface of mandible	Upper border of hyoid bone	Trigeminal	Elevates tongue and floor of mouth, depresses jaw when hyoid bone is in fixed position
Digastric (anterior belly)	Intermediate tendon by loop of fascia to hyoid bone	Lower border of mandible	Trigeminal	Raises hyoid bone if jaw is in fixed position, depresses jaw if hyoid bone is in fixed position
Geniohyoid	Mental spine of mandible	Hyoid bone	Cervical (C1 and C2) through hypoglossal	Draws hyoid bone forward, depresses mandible when hyoid bone is in fixed position
Stylohyoid	Styloid process of temporal bone	Body of hyoid at greater cornu	Facial	Elevates hyoid and tongue base
Hyoglossus	Greater cornu of hyoid	Into tongue sides	Hypoglossal	Tongue depression
Genioglossus	Upper genial tubercle of mandible	Hyoid, inferior tongue, and tip	Hypoglossal	Protrusion and depression
Styloglossus	Anterior border of styloid process	Into side of tongue	Hypoglossal	Elevates up and back
Palatoglossus	Anterior surface of soft palate	Dorsum and side of tongue	Glossopharyngeal, vagus, and accessory	Narrows fauces and elevates posterior tongue

Table 1.4.   Muscles of the Soft Palate.

Muscle	Origin	Insertion	Nerve	Action
Levator veli palatini	Apex of temporal bone	Palatine aponeurosis of soft palate	Vagus and accessory	Raises soft palate
Tensor veli palatini	Fossa of sphenoid bone	Palatine aponeurosis of soft palate	Trigeminal	Stretches soft palate
Palatoglossus	Undersurface of soft palate	Side of tongue	Vagus and accessory	Raises back of tongue during first stage of swallowing
Palatopharyngeus	Soft palate	Pharyngeal wall	Vagus and accessory	Shuts off nasopharynx during second stage of swallowing
Uvular	Posterior nasal spine and palatine aponeurosis	Into uvula to form its chief bulk or content	Vagus and accessory	Shortens and raises uvula

The cricopharyngeus muscle is an important single muscle that lies at the transition level between pharynx and esophagus. Functionally, it is separate from both the pharynx and esophagus and acts as a sphincter, relaxing during passage of the bolus from the pharynx into the esophagus. Although its innervation is somewhat controversial, it is probably innervated by both the pharyngeal branch of the vagus and the recurrent laryngeal branch of the vagus.

Sequence of Movements and Phenomena of Normal Swallowing

Healthy persons simultaneously perform many acts involving the sequential steps of chewing and swallowing. Most of these only are minimally conscious, even though voluntary, yet they depend on highly intricate coordination. Thus a single bolus of varying texture and taste can be chewed and swallowed while the person carries on a conversation, and at the same time a beverage may be imbibed while one holds various portions of the more solid texture in the mouth with relatively little awareness or concentration. As is discussed in connection with neurologic disorders of swallowing (see Chapter 2), ab-

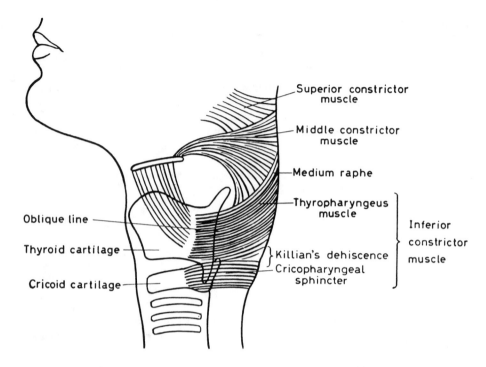

Figure 1.4. The muscular pharynx. Reprinted by permission of the publisher, from Ballantyne and Groves, 1971.

normalities of the oropharyngeal mechanism in particular may result in increased awareness of, and attention devoted to, the entire act of swallowing.

Food introduced into the mouth cannot be prepared for swallowing by being formed into a bolus unless it is mixed with saliva contributed from three pairs of major salivary glands. The parotid gland receives parasympathetic nerve supply by way of the glossopharyngeal nerve from the inferior salivary nucleus located in the lower brainstem. The submandibular and sublingual glands are innervated by parasympathetic fibers of the facial nerve. Each gland has single or multiple excretory ducts opening into the mouth.

The usual conditions associated with normal swallowing are a moist cavity, open nostrils, and a closed mouth. The steps involved are illustrated in Figure 1.5. As a bolus is masticated, the tongue tip is elevated to occlude the anterior oral cavity at the alveolar ridge and the bolus is compressed against the hard palate. This is a preparatory position in which the posterior portion of the tongue has maneuvered the bolus into position. As swallowing begins, the anterior portion of the tongue is retracted and depressed, mastication then ceases, and respiration is reflexly inhibited. Retraction of the tongue and elevation against the hard palate force the bolus into the upper part of the pharynx. The palatopharyngeal folds are pulled medially to form a slit through which properly masticated food can pass. The levator and

Table 1.5.   Muscles of the Pharynx.

Muscle	Origin	Insertion	Nerve	Action
Palatopha-ryngeus	Extends from soft palate to pharyngeal wall	Posterior border of thyroid cartilage and pharyngeal aponeurosis	Pharyngeal plexus and accessory	Narrows oropharynx, elevates pharynx, shuts off nasopharynx
Stylopharyn-geus	Medial side of root of styloid process	Superior and inferior borders of thyroid cartilage	Glossopharyngeal	Raises and dilates pharynx
Salpingo-pharyngeus	Pharyngeal end of auditory tube	Blends with palatopharyngeus	Pharyngeal plexus and accessory	Raises nasopharynx, draws lateral pharyngeal walls up

tensor veli palatini muscles help to elevate the soft palate and block the nasopharyngeal opening.

The pharyngeal stage begins with movements of the tongue posteriorly to drive the bolus into the pharynx while the entire larynx is pulled upward and forward. This action causes the epiglottis to approximate the base of the tongue, which blocks and protects the airway (see sequence in Figure 1.5). Food is directed to either side of the epiglottis. Further protection during this reflexive stage is provided when respiration has ceased, allowing the vocal cords to close off the trachea. In preparation for propulsion of food toward the esophagus, the cricopharyngeus relaxes and is pulled open in contrast to its sympathetically induced tonic contraction as an esophageal sphincter. Relaxation is accomplished by parasympathetic impulses over the vagus nerve, along with passive opening of the sphincter by laryngeal elevation and tilting. The bolus is propelled into the esophagus, again by a "stripping" action accomplished by the pharyngeal constrictors.

In the esophageal phase, the bolus is carried toward the stomach by gravity and peristalsis. The latter begins in the pharynx and spreads into the body of the esophagus toward the lower sphincter proximal to the stomach, an action that is supplemented by secondary waves.

A more detailed account of the neural regulation of deglutition is presented later in this chapter. Thus far, we have seen that both the central nervous system and the autonomic nervous system exert a balance of excitation and inhibition resulting in a highly coordinated and integrated contraction of certain muscles in phase with simultaneous relaxation of other muscle groups.

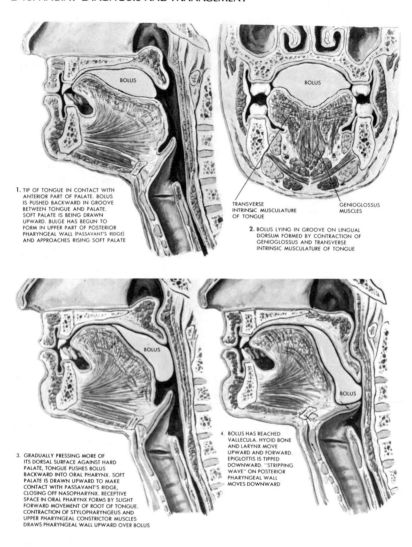

1. TIP OF TONGUE IN CONTACT WITH ANTERIOR PART OF PALATE. BOLUS IS PUSHED BACKWARD IN GROOVE BETWEEN TONGUE AND PALATE. SOFT PALATE IS BEING DRAWN UPWARD. BULGE HAS BEGUN TO FORM IN UPPER PART OF POSTERIOR PHARYNGEAL WALL (PASSAVANT'S RIDGE) AND APPROACHES RISING SOFT PALATE

2. BOLUS LYING IN GROOVE ON LINGUAL DORSUM FORMED BY CONTRACTION OF GENIOGLOSSUS AND TRANSVERSE INTRINSIC MUSCULATURE OF TONGUE

TRANSVERSE INTRINSIC MUSCULATURE OF TONGUE

GENIOGLOSSUS MUSCLES

3. GRADUALLY PRESSING MORE OF ITS DORSAL SURFACE AGAINST HARD PALATE, TONGUE PUSHES BOLUS BACKWARD INTO ORAL PHARYNX. SOFT PALATE IS DRAWN UPWARD TO MAKE CONTACT WITH PASSAVANT'S RIDGE, CLOSING OFF NASOPHARYNX. RECEPTIVE SPACE IN ORAL PHARYNX FORMS BY SLIGHT FORWARD MOVEMENT OF ROOT OF TONGUE. CONTRACTION OF STYLOPHARYNGEUS AND UPPER PHARYNGEAL CONSTRICTOR MUSCLES DRAWS PHARYNGEAL WALL UPWARD OVER BOLUS

4. BOLUS HAS REACHED VALLECULA. HYOID BONE AND LARYNX MOVE UPWARD AND FORWARD. EPIGLOTTIS IS TIPPED DOWNWARD. "STRIPPING WAVE" ON POSTERIOR PHARYNGEAL WALL MOVES DOWNWARD

Figure 1.5.   Sequential presentation of the steps involved in the normal swallow. © Copyright 1959, CIBA Pharmaceutical Company, Division of CIBA-GEIGY Corporation. Reprinted with permission, from THE CIBA COLLECTION OF MEDICAL ILLUSTRATIONS, illustrated by Frank H. Netter, M.D. All rights reserved.

The essential physiologic requirements for deglutition consist of the following: (1) development of a bolus, (2) prevention of disbursal of the bolus throughout swallowing, (3) development of differential pressures allowing bolus propulsion, (4) prevention of entrance of food or fluid into the nasopharynx and larynx, (5) rapid transit of the bolus through the pharynx to minimize the suspension of respiration, (6) prevention of gastric reflux during esophageal emptying, and (7) clearing of residual material from the

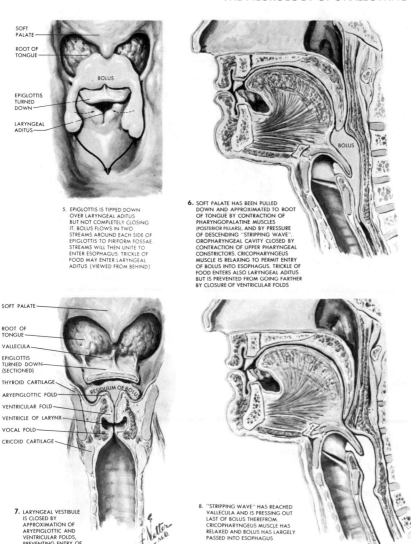

SOFT
PALATE

ROOT OF
TONGUE

BOLUS

EPIGLOTTIS
TURNED
DOWN

LARYNGEAL
ADITUS

BOLUS

5. EPIGLOTTIS IS TIPPED DOWN
OVER LARYNGEAL ADITUS
BUT NOT COMPLETELY CLOSING
IT. BOLUS FLOWS IN TWO
STREAMS AROUND EACH SIDE OF
EPIGLOTTIS TO PIRIFORM FOSSAE
STREAMS WILL THEN UNITE TO
ENTER ESOPHAGUS. TRICKLE OF
FOOD MAY ENTER LARYNGEAL
ADITUS (VIEWED FROM BEHIND)

6. SOFT PALATE HAS BEEN PULLED
DOWN AND APPROXIMATED TO ROOT
OF TONGUE BY CONTRACTION OF
PHARYNGOPALATINE MUSCLES
(POSTERIOR PILLARS), AND BY PRESSURE
OF DESCENDING "STRIPPING WAVE".
OROPHARYNGEAL CAVITY CLOSED BY
CONTRACTION OF UPPER PHARYNGEAL
CONSTRICTORS. CRICOPHARYNGEUS
MUSCLE IS RELAXING TO PERMIT ENTRY
OF BOLUS INTO ESOPHAGUS. TRICKLE OF
FOOD ENTERS ALSO LARYNGEAL ADITUS
BUT IS PREVENTED FROM GOING FARTHER
BY CLOSURE OF VENTRICULAR FOLDS

SOFT PALATE

ROOT OF
TONGUE

VALLECULA

EPIGLOTTIS
TURNED DOWN
(SECTIONED)

THYROID CARTILAGE

ARYEPIGLOTTIC FOLD

VENTRICULAR FOLD

VENTRICLE OF LARYNX

VOCAL FOLD

CRICOID CARTILAGE

RESIDUUM OF BOLUS

7. LARYNGEAL VESTIBULE
IS CLOSED BY
APPROXIMATION OF
ARYEPIGLOTTIC AND
VENTRICULAR FOLDS,
PREVENTING ENTRY
OF FOOD INTO LARYNX
(CORONAL SECTION:
A-P VIEW)

8. "STRIPPING WAVE" HAS REACHED
VALLECULA AND IS PRESSING OUT
LAST OF BOLUS THEREFROM.
CRICOPHARYNGEUS MUSCLE HAS
RELAXED AND BOLUS HAS LARGELY
PASSED INTO ESOPHAGUS

F. Netter
M.D.
© CIBA

Figure 1.5.   *(continued)*

pharyngoesophageal tract. Since so many important and functionally separate changes occur during a short period of time in the swallowing mechanism, it will be helpful to review the sequence with emphasis on other aspects that relate to the three primary stages previously outlined.

The following numerical sequence is taken from Donner and Siegel (1965) as revised and extended by Donner (1974): (1) tongue movements that initiate the act of swallowing require concomitant contraction of mylohyoid, geniohyoid, and digastric muscles in the floor of the mouth; (2) the

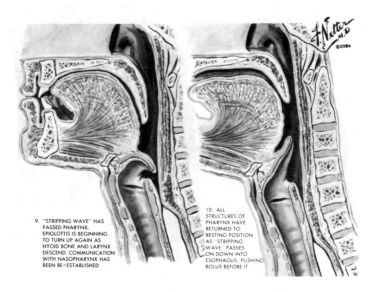

9. "STRIPPING WAVE" HAS PASSED PHARYNX. EPIGLOTTIS IS BEGINNING TO TURN UP AGAIN AS HYOID BONE AND LARYNX DESCEND. COMMUNICATION WITH NASOPHARYNX HAS BEEN RE−ESTABLISHED

10. ALL STRUCTURES OF PHARYNX HAVE RETURNED TO RESTING POSITION AS "STRIPPING WAVE" PASSES ON DOWN INTO ESOPHAGUS, PUSHING BOLUS BEFORE IT

Figure 1.5.   *(continued)*

styloglossus and hyoglossus muscles force the root of the tongue against the soft palate and posterior pharyngeal wall; (3) the levator and tensor veli palatini muscles elevate the soft palate, with additional shortening and dorsal thickening until approximation against the posterior pharyngeal muscle prevents nasopharyngeal regurgitation; (4) the middle and inferior pharyngeal constrictor muscles narrow the hypopharynx and contribute to the peristaltic movements involving the posterior pharyngeal wall, which generally are located between the level of Passavant's cushion and the cricopharyngeal sphincter; and (5) dorsal and downward tilting of the epiglottis is brought about by the muscular elevation of the larynx and contraction of the floor of the mouth with concomitant elevation and posterior movement of the hyoid bone. Neuromuscular disorders easily affect the highly coordinated physiologic swallowing process that delicately adjusts opening of the cricopharynx and closure of the trachea as food passes the pharynx under circumstances in which the pharynx will be freed from food when the airway again opens. The five sequential steps outlined are keyed in Figure 1.6. Among the detailed studies on oropharyngeal movements during swallowing, useful articles are those by Ardran and Kemp (1951) and Sloan et al. (1964).

Laryngeal Stage of Swallowing

The bolus is sucked into the laryngopharynx by the production of a zone of negative pressure, occurring when the upward movement of hyoid and larynx are coupled with the forward and posterior tilting motion of the latter. This creates a pulling force and increases the anteroposterior diameter of the laryngopharynx.

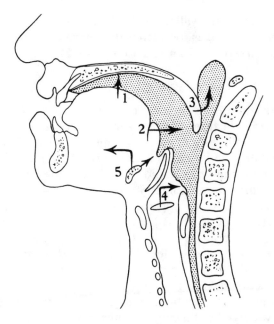

Figure 1.6.   Summary of the five important
physiologic events involved in the normal
swallow. Reprinted by permission of the publisher from Donner, *American Journal of
Roentgenology,* vol. 94, © 1965.

Contraction of intrinsic laryngeal muscles shortens and widens the aryepiglottic folds and vocal and vestibular folds, producing an airtight soft
stopper for the subglottic region. This eliminates the departure of air from
the respiratory tract, which would oppose a sucking effect. The laryngeal
ventricles probably are obliterated at this point while the epiglottis moves
downward and backward as a result of approximation of the thyroid cartilage
to the hyoid bone. Epiglottic depression does not completely close the laryngeal aditus, a result of which is the insertion of small particles of the bolus
into that opening for a short distance.

A liquid bolus is usually split by the epiglottis, traveling on each side
of the larynx through the pyriform recesses to rejoin behind the cricoid
cartilage (see Figure 1.2). The epiglottis acts as a ledge, checking the descent
of the bolus and obviating early closure of the larynx. Protection of the
larynx during swallowing is effected in part by closure due to contraction of
the sphincteric girdle of muscle that surrounds it. This occurs without elevation of the larynx. The larynx may be closed at any stage during swallowing
but is always closed when the last of the bolus leaves the pharynx, at which
point material entering the vestibule of the larynx is squeezed out. The hood
formed by the epiglottis bending downward over the entrance to the larynx
prevents the deposition of a residue, and reinflation of the airway carries

any residue upward into the vallecula. In the absence of epiglottic function, repeated swallowing removes food from the entrance to the larynx prior to reinflation of the airway (Ardran and Kemp, 1952).

Normal Function of the Esophagus

Esophageal tasks require an ordered pattern of function that depends on coordinated activities in three distinct zones: esophageal inlet, esophageal outlet, and body of the esophagus. The inlet consists of visceral striated muscle that maintains the lumen in a closed position and is integrated with the tongue and hypopharynx. Rapid events here are analyzed by cineradiography or intraluminal manometry (see Chapter 4). The high-pressure zone, which is equivalent to an upper esophageal sphincter, relaxes promptly on swallowing during a period timed to coincide with pharyngeal contraction and movement of the bolus into the upper end of the esophagus. In the esophageal outlet, the lumen is closed by specialized muscle that is distinguished from the body of the esophagus and separates it from the stomach. Only during the act of swallowing does the pressure in this zone fall, but a gradient is maintained between the esophagus and stomach so that the lumen does not open widely. Swallowing initiates a moving contraction that is ringlike and sweeps rapidly through the upper striated portion and less rapidly through the lower smooth muscle portion. The terminal portion or outlet that is located about 1 to 2 cm above the diaphragm is referred to as the gastroesophageal vestibule or high-pressure zone. Evacuation of the vestibule filled from above inhibits reflux of the stomach's content into the esophagus and thus functions as a valve. Proximal to this vestibule is a functional ampulla, which serves as a collecting area where pressure is built by the peristaltic wave moving toward it (Figure 1.7). Further details concerning the methodology and applications of intraluminal esophageal manometry may be found in Dodds (1976), Castell (1980), and Chapter 4 of this volume.

NEURAL REGULATION OF SWALLOWING

Overview

Swallowing usually is initiated by sensory impulses transmitted as a result of stimulation of receptors on the fauces, tonsils, soft palate, base of the tongue, and posterior pharyngeal wall. These sensory impulses reach the brainstem primarily through the seventh, ninth, and tenth cranial nerves, while the efferent function is mediated through the ninth, tenth, and twelfth cranial nerves (see Tables 1.6 and 1.7). Cricopharyngeal sphincter opening is reflexive, relaxation occurring at the time when the bolus reaches the posterior pharyngeal wall prior to reaching this sphincter.

Although reference is made in the literature to a so-called swallowing

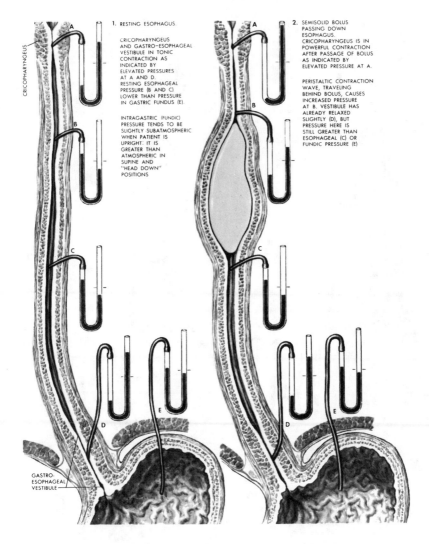

CRICOPHARYNGEUS

1. RESTING ESOPHAGUS.

CRICOPHARYNGEUS
AND GASTRO-ESOPHAGEAL
VESTIBULE IN TONIC
CONTRACTION AS
INDICATED BY
ELEVATED PRESSURES
AT A AND D.
RESTING ESOPHAGEAL
PRESSURE (B AND C)
LOWER THAN PRESSURE
IN GASTRIC FUNDUS (E).

INTRAGASTRIC (FUNDIC)
PRESSURE TENDS TO BE
SLIGHTLY SUBATMOSPHERIC
WHEN PATIENT IS
UPRIGHT. IT IS
GREATER THAN
ATMOSPHERIC IN
SUPINE AND
"HEAD DOWN"
POSITIONS

2. SEMISOLID BOLUS
PASSING DOWN
ESOPHAGUS.
CRICOPHARYNGEUS IS IN
POWERFUL CONTRACTION
AFTER PASSAGE OF BOLUS
AS INDICATED BY
ELEVATED PRESSURE AT A.

PERISTALTIC CONTRACTION
WAVE, TRAVELING
BEHIND BOLUS, CAUSES
INCREASED PRESSURE
AT B. VESTIBULE HAS
ALREADY RELAXED
SLIGHTLY (D), BUT
PRESSURE HERE IS
STILL GREATER THAN
ESOPHAGEAL (C) OR
FUNDIC PRESSURE (E)

GASTRO-
ESOPHAGEAL
VESTIBULE

Figure 1.7.   Pressure relationships above and below the esophagus that regulate portions of gastroesophageal functioning. © Copyright 1959, CIBA Pharmaceutical Company, Division of CIBA-GEIGY Corporation. Reprinted with permission, from THE CIBA COLLECTION OF MEDICAL ILLUSTRATIONS, illustrated by Frank H. Netter, M.D. All rights reserved.

center, this is probably an oversimplification and it is likely that modulation of the swallowing function and its coordinated mechanisms result from impulse activity in cranial nerves other than those intermittently associated with the swallowing itself. An example would be the fifth cranial nerve. In ad-

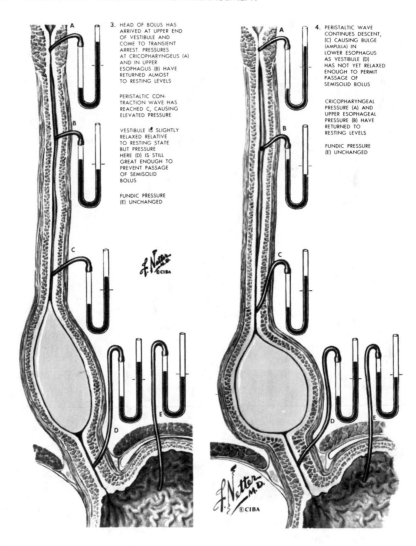

3. HEAD OF BOLUS HAS ARRIVED AT UPPER END OF VESTIBULE AND COME TO TRANSIENT ARREST. PRESSURES AT CRICOPHARYNGEUS (A) AND IN UPPER ESOPHAGUS (B) HAVE RETURNED ALMOST TO RESTING LEVELS

PERISTALTIC CONTRACTION WAVE HAS REACHED C, CAUSING ELEVATED PRESSURE

VESTIBULE IS SLIGHTLY RELAXED RELATIVE TO RESTING STATE BUT PRESSURE HERE (D) IS STILL GREAT ENOUGH TO PREVENT PASSAGE OF SEMISOLID BOLUS

FUNDIC PRESSURE (E) UNCHANGED

4. PERISTALTIC WAVE CONTINUES DESCENT, (C) CAUSING BULGE (AMPULLA) IN LOWER ESOPHAGUS AS VESTIBULE (D) HAS NOT YET RELAXED ENOUGH TO PERMIT PASSAGE OF SEMISOLID BOLUS

CRICOPHARYNGEAL PRESSURE (A) AND UPPER ESOPHAGEAL PRESSURE (B) HAVE RETURNED TO RESTING LEVELS

FUNDIC PRESSURE (E) UNCHANGED

Figure 1.7.   *(continued)*

dition, salivatory preparation of the bolus cannot occur in the absence of cholinergic activity mediated through the peripheral and autonomic nervous systems. The striated muscle mediating swallowing in the pharynx, cricopharyngeal sphincter, and upper one-third of the esophagus are under the control of impulses originating in motoneurons of the corresponding cranial nerve nuclei. The smooth muscular structures associated with swallowing, however, are innervated by cholinergic vagal preganglionic fibers that synapse with a plexus in the muscle itself; for example, the wall of the esophagus, resulting in postganglionic release of acetylcholine.

The upper esophageal sphincter adjacent to the cricopharyngeus is under control of the nucleus ambiguus and the dorsal motor nucleus of the

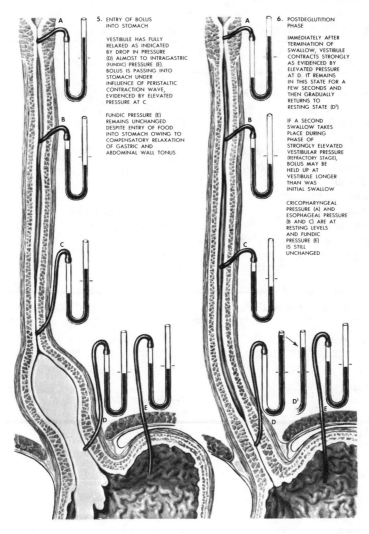

5. ENTRY OF BOLUS INTO STOMACH

VESTIBULE HAS FULLY RELAXED AS INDICATED BY DROP IN PRESSURE (D) ALMOST TO INTRAGASTRIC (FUNDIC) PRESSURE (E). BOLUS IS PASSING INTO STOMACH UNDER INFLUENCE OF PERISTALTIC CONTRACTION WAVE, EVIDENCED BY ELEVATED PRESSURE AT C

FUNDIC PRESSURE (E) REMAINS UNCHANGED DESPITE ENTRY OF FOOD INTO STOMACH OWING TO COMPENSATORY RELAXATION OF GASTRIC AND ABDOMINAL WALL TONUS

6. POSTDEGLUTITION PHASE

IMMEDIATELY AFTER TERMINATION OF SWALLOW, VESTIBULE CONTRACTS STRONGLY AS EVIDENCED BY ELEVATED PRESSURE AT D. IT REMAINS IN THIS STATE FOR A FEW SECONDS AND THEN GRADUALLY RETURNS TO RESTING STATE (D¹)

IF A SECOND SWALLOW TAKES PLACE DURING PHASE OF STRONGLY ELEVATED VESTIBULAR PRESSURE (REFRACTORY STAGE), BOLUS MAY BE HELD UP AT VESTIBULE LONGER THAN WAS INITIAL SWALLOW

CRICOPHARYNGEAL PRESSURE (A) AND ESOPHAGEAL PRESSURE (B AND C) ARE AT RESTING LEVELS AND FUNDIC PRESSURE (E) IS STILL UNCHANGED

Figure 1.7. *(continued)*

tenth cranial nerve. The lower esophageal sphincter relates to thickened bands of muscle in the diaphragmatic hiatus, and is at least partially under vagal control. The extrinsic esophageal musculature is under influence of the vagus nerve and the sympathetic nervous system (cervical and thoracic ganglia) with intrinsic neuroramifications by way of the plexuses of Auerbach and Meissner (parasympathetic postganglionic neurons in submucosal layer of gastrointestinal tract). There is some controversy over the origin of the cricopharyngeal resting tone, which may not rely solely on the sympathetic nervous system, but may be more heavily dependent upon vagal input, both for contraction and for relaxation (Palmer, 1976).

Table 1.6. Afferent Controls Involved in Swallowing.

Sensory Function	Innervation
General sensation, anterior two-thirds of tongue	Lingual nerve, trigeminal (V)
Taste, anterior two-thirds tongue	Chorda tympani, facial (VII)
Taste and general sensation, posterior one-third of the tongue	Glossopharyngeal (IX)
Mucosa of vallecula	Internal branch of SLN (vagus)
Primary afferent	Glossopharyngeal (IX)
Secondary afferent	Pharyngeal branch of vagus (X)
Tonsils, pharynx, soft palate	Glossopharyngeal (IX)
Pharynx, larynx, viscera	Vagus (X)

Table 1.7. Efferent Controls Involved in Swallowing.

Efferent/Stage	Innervation
Oral	
Masticatory, buccinator, floor of mouth	Trigeminal (V)
Lip sphincter	Facial (VII)
Tongue	Hypoglossal (XII)
Pharyngeal	
Constrictors and stylopharyngeus	Glossopharyngeal (IX)
Palate, pharynx, larynx	Vagus (X)
Tongue	Hypoglossal (XII)
Esophageal	
Esophagus	Vagus (X)

Neuromuscular Elements and Coordinated Nerve Supply in Normal Swallowing

The highly integrated activities of swallowing depend on a combination of voluntary and involuntary control of the position of lips, teeth, jaw, cheeks, and tongue, all partly mediated by the fifth cranial nerve-innervated muscles that control both the mandible and the masseter. Both of these muscles are involved in the control of leverage, stabilization, and centering of the movable parts of the buccal cavity. Therefore, mastication depends primarily on the fifth cranial nerve, whereas the muscles of the lips and cheeks depend on motor functions of the seventh cranial nerve. All of the extrinsic muscles of the tongue depend on the motor function of the twelfth cranial nerve, except for the palatoglossus (elevator of the tongue root), which is innervated by the tenth cranial nerve. All of the intrinsic lingual muscles are innervated by the twelfth cranial nerve. All of the muscles of the soft palate are innervated primarily by the tenth cranial nerve, except the tensor veli palatini, which is innervated by the fifth cranial nerve. The stylopharyngeus, a longitudinal muscle, has the function of widening the pharynx and is innervated by the ninth cranial nerve, whereas the palatopharyngeus is innervated primarily by the tenth cranial nerve. The maxillary and mandibular sensory divisions of the fifth cranial nerve are primarily involved in providing sensation pertaining to the lips, palate, teeth, inner mouth, and proprioceptive aspects of the muscles of mastication. The gag reflex as well as nasal regurgitation depends on the function or dysfunction of the glossopharyngeal and vagus nerves, whose muscles of innervation have been discussed previously. The characteristics of upper and lower motoneuron lesions of some of the more important cranial nerves subserving deglutition are discussed in Chapter 2.

The voluntary components of swallowing probably have their origin in higher cerebral centers, some of which have been localized. They operate primarily upon striated muscles, but involve the development of "automatisms" that still may be subject to voluntary monitoring and control, although they appear to be involuntary. These include the "habits" of mouth control and chewing, which are largely distinguishable from individual to individual. Many of the neuromechanisms dependent on combination of the pathways referred to above combine in complex reflexes other than swallowing, such as cough and gag, and others that have variable expression at different stages of life. Examples include the rooting and sucking of infancy, and the biting reflexes dependent on masseteric stretch.

At the cortical level, the inferior portion of the precentral gyrus of the insula produces swallowing movements on electrical stimulation. These may result from efferent connections to the hypothalamus and thence to the medulla where the so-called swallowing center has been identified (in the region of the ala cinerea [4th ventricle] and the tenth cranial nerve nuclei).

The Swallowing Center

The swallowing center coordinates efferent impulse flow by way of the fifth, tenth, and twelfth cranial nerves to the levators (soft palate), by way of the tenth cranial nerve to the pharyngeal constrictors, through the cervical and thoracic spinal nerves to the diaphragm and intercostals, by way of the fifth and twelfth cranial nerves to the extrinsic muscles of the larynx, and by way of the tenth cranial nerve to the intrinsic muscles of the larynx and esophagus. The cervical esophagus may receive two efferent supplies: one from the recurrent laryngeal and another from the pharyngoesophageal nerve that rises proximal to the nodose ganglion (inferior to jugular foramen), or from an esophageal branch of the external laryngeal portion of the superior laryngeal nerve (SLN). Double innervation in man has not been proved, but might provide a margin of safety.

Sequentially timed discharges from the medullary center mediate the movement of a bolus through successive levels of the esophageal musculature. A sequence of esophageal contractions appears to include a mechanism by which proximal activity inhibits the next most distal portion of the esophagus successively. Esophageal distention is signaled on visceral efferent nerves passing in the upper five or six thoracic sympathetic roots, presumably to the thalamus and inferior postcentral gyrus where they may give rise to symptoms described as pressure, burning, gas, aching, and the like. When such symptoms are described as pain, the referral patterns are based on sensory impulses from tissues innervated by somatic nerves that cross the corresponding spinal levels.

Because of the widespread ramifications and functional significance of the vagus nerve (tenth), lesions in the vagal system may have far-reaching deleterious effects on coughing, swallowing, breathing, and phonation, elements of each of which are interrelated at various vagal levels. Although the details of anatomic and physiologic complexity are beyond the scope of this discussion, it is essential that the reader grasp the major pattern of vagal distribution (Figure 1.8). Swallowing is a lower-level response, yet its afferent side can be stimulated by voluntary movements of the tongue and larynx. This is subserved to some extent by separation of corticobulbar fibers, with some remaining ipsilateral and some providing contralateral innervation to the nucleus ambiguus (motor ninth and tenth). The latter forms the brainstem locus from which special visceral efferent fibers arise. Cerebral centers that may be associated with the representation of swallowing also appear to produce phonation or vocal fold adduction by way of extrapyramidal, multi-synaptic connections that are completely separate from the precentral swallowing locus of area 4.

Fibers originating in the nucleus ambiguus innervate the pharyngeal, laryngeal, and upper esophageal striated muscles. The vagus nerve itself is formed from dorsal efferent and inferior salivatory nuclei. It also innervates the heart, lungs, and gastrointestinal tract smooth muscle. It carries afferents for taste, pharyngeal sensation, and sensation from some regions of skin around the external ear. Rootlets emerging from the brainstem form the peripheral vagus, which exits the skull through the jugular foramen. Above the nodose ganglion, the vagus nerve sends branches to the pharyngeal plexus, which supplies the mucosa and musculature of the pharynx, larynx, and upper esophagus. At this point it is accompanied by branches from the neighboring sympathetic ganglia.

The very important superior laryngeal nerve (SLN) is sensory to the laryngeal mucosa and motor to the cricothyroid muscle. The vagus terminates

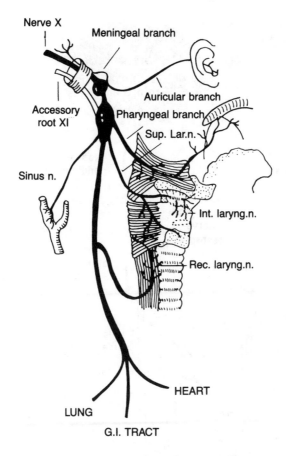

Figure 1.8. Course of the peripheral vagus nerve on exit from the jugular foramen. Reprinted by permission of the publisher, from Rontal and Rontal, *Laryngoscope,* vol. 87, no. 1, January 1977.

as the recurrent laryngeal nerve that loops around the aorta and returns to the larynx and hypopharynx (Figure 1.9). The recurrent laryngeal nerve supplies muscles intrinsic to the larynx and is thought not to supply the cricopharyngeus, which apparently derives its innervation from the pharyngeal plexus. Clinical aspects of disorders affecting various levels of the vagus nerve are discussed in Chapter 2.

Neural Control Systems Subserving Swallowing

The neural control systems that subserve swallowing differ somewhat from the fundamental anatomic arrangements discussed in the preceding section.

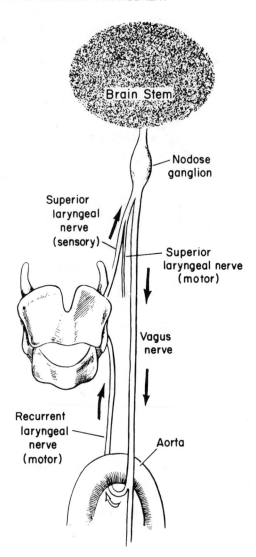

Figure 1.9. The reflex arc responsible for laryngeal closure consists of the sensory limb of the vagus (superior laryngeal nerve) and the motor limb of the vagus (recurrent laryngeal nerve). Note how the vagus terminates inferiorly around the aorta, returning to the larynx and hypopharynx. Reprinted by permission of the publisher, from Sasaki, Paralysis of the larynx and pharynx, *Surgical Clinics of North America,* 60:1079–92, 1980.

These control systems include a buccopharyngeal, an esophageal, and a gastroesophageal phase which, through appropriate coordinated activity, result in the normal sequence of events but can function as separate entities. Once set in motion, some of the sequential events continue, regardless of afferent activity. Others may depend in varying degrees upon efferent or supranuclear activity. Esophageal function is alterable by afferent feedback. While some of the specifics of the control mechanisms for these systems remain controversial, the discussion considers those aspects that are accepted more fully.

It appears that swallowing can be initiated by the action of peripheral afferents alone, but that isolated central activation is not possible even though voluntary components exist. The widespread competent afferent system and its distribution have been described. If a concept of a swallowing center is accepted, then it appears that afferent impulses competent to initiate swallowing must conform to highly codified stimulus patterns that enter the nucleus solitarius of the brainstem by way of its fasciculus and are relayed into the reticular formation where connections exist to motoneurons lying in the nuclei of the fifth, seventh, and twelfth cranial nerves and the nucleus ambiguus. These neurons are interesting in that they lack recurrent collaterals or monosynaptic connections and apparently do not connect disynaptically with peripheral afferents. The motoneurons for the smooth muscle part of the esophagus appear to be located in the dorsal motor nucleus of the tenth cranial nerve.

The swallowing center is the basis of the buccopharyngeal component of swallowing and exists within the medullary reticular formation, 1.5 mm from the midline on either side, and 1 to 3 mm posterior to the inferior olive between the anterior end of the inferior olive and the caudal or inferior end of the facial nucleus. On each side of the midline exists a half-center that communicates with the opposite half-center through cross connections running behind the obex or through the trapezoid body. As a result, bilateral symmetry of swallowing action is achieved. Each half-center exerts ipsilateral inhibition on appropriate motoneurons, although excitatory action may also be strictly ipsilateral with the exception of excitation to the lower constrictor muscles, which are strictly contralateral (Figure 1.10).

The buccopharyngeal component involves a sequence of excitation and inhibition produced by several motoneuronal pools on each side of the brainstem. Through chronologic synergy that can be reproduced electrically by stimulation of the internal branch of the SLN, the esophageal and gastroesophageal components follow. From an electrophysiologic standpoint, swallowing probably is the most complex behavioral pattern that can be evoked by electrical stimulation of a peripheral nerve. Since normal swallowing occurs in humans who congenitally have no neural tissue rostral to the red nucleus, and in experimental animals whose brain is intact at least caudally from the motor nucleus of the tenth cranial nerve, its control appears not to depend unequivocally on cerebral structures or on the cerebellum or

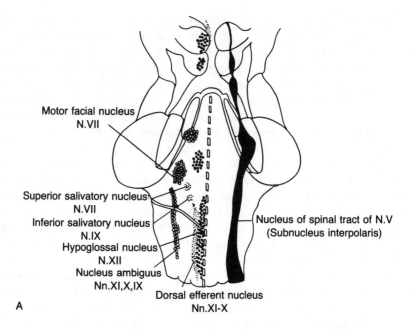

Motor facial nucleus
N.VII

Superior salivatory nucleus
N.VII
Inferior salivatory nucleus
N.IX
Hypoglossal nucleus
N.XII
Nucleus ambiguus
Nn.XI,X,IX

Nucleus of spinal tract of N.V
(Subnucleus interpolaris)

Dorsal efferent nucleus
Nn.XI-X

A

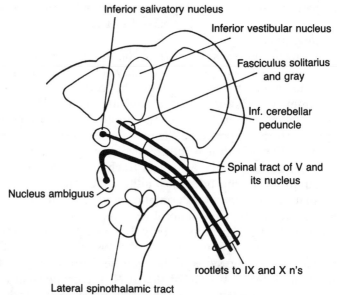

Inferior salivatory nucleus

Inferior vestibular nucleus

Fasciculus solitarius
and gray

Inf. cerebellar
peduncle

Spinal tract of V and
its nucleus

Nucleus ambiguus

rootlets to IX and X n's

B   Lateral spinothalamic tract

Figure 1.10. (A) Longitudinal section through the medulla showing relationships of the vagus nerve to the surrounding structures (after Crosby). (B) Cross section at the level of the medulla showing relationship of the vagus nerve to the surrounding structures (after Crosby). Reprinted by permission of the publisher, from Rontal and Rontal, *Laryngoscope,* vol. 87, no. 1, January 1977.

inferior olives. It appears also that some form of bolus is necessary to sustain repetitive swallowing, a fact that highlights the importance of peripheral stimuli.

The neural organization of swallowing has been largely elucidated by recording the electrical activity of involved muscles, beginning with onset of contraction in the mylohyoid and including concurrent activity in muscles innervated by the fifth cranial nerve and those of the posterior tongue, superior constrictor, palatopharyngeus, palatoglossus, stylohyoid, and geniohyoid. These initiators constitute what has been called the leading complex (Doty and Bosma, 1956). Since the constrictors form a continuous sheet of striated muscle, an overlapping firing sequence is observed, beginning with the pterygopharyngeus or superior constrictor (the principle muscle), the hypopharyngeus or middle constrictor, and the inferior constrictor with distinct rostral (thyropharyngeus) and caudal (cricopharyngeus) components. The superior constrictor is active at the same time as the leading complex activity. A reconstruction of firing patterns leads to the conclusion that inhibition would probably be found to surround or bracket (in a time sense) the excitation of swallowing.

The neural structures and organization of swallowing result in more than one basic type of swallowing pattern, for example, that found in infancy, and more mature patterns developing later in childhood, adolescence, and adulthood. There also is variation from individual to individual. Some believe that these may be imposed by higher centers, but an alternative is that there is variable organization of the swallowing center itself.

At the pharyngoesophageal junction, the upper movement of the larynx may be functionally related to the opening of the passive elastic sphincter. This movement may be assisted by the activity of the geniohyoid muscles. Closure of the pharyngoesophageal junction probably occurs normally by passive elasticity of surrounding tissues, but more than one kind of reflex exists that can contract the cricopharyngeus. This contraction, however, is prevented by activity in the swallowing center that inhibits cricopharyngeal motoneurons.

A fundamental description of the neuroregulation of swallowing requires a somewhat artificial isolation of the neural organization. Actually, movements of the palate and swallowing are probably closely related to those occurring in speech and respiration. Earlier evolutionary patterns such as swallowing of air by amphibia may be regained by adult humans, for example, victims of poliomyelitis. Such movements require some voluntary control of the inferior constrictor with pumping tongue movements, suggestive of glossopharyngeal breathing.

From the standpoint of peripheral innervation, elicitation of swallowing may occur as a result of activity in the maxillary branch of the trigeminal, glossopharyngeal, or SLN. It has been suggested that small fibers giving rise to a superficial plexus of beaded terminals on the pharyngeal surface of the epiglottis may be the type of nerve ending that is most likely to be activated in the initiation of swallowing. Many complex endings also exist on the oral side of the soft palate or uvula, although anatomic complexity and overlap make it difficult to identify elements specifically at this point. In addition to sensory endings, there are proprioceptors whose relevance to swallowing has not been clarified. It is important that there probably are not more than 2,000 motoneurons on both sides to innervate about 12,000 constrictor muscle fibers, and that this low innervation ratio of the pharyngeal musculature implies neural control comparable in precision to that of the ocular muscles.

CENTRAL CONTROL OF SWALLOWING

It is necessary to deal in more detail with the central afferent systems, the motoneuron pools, and the efferent systems, since the localization of central organization of swallowing (swallowing center) could be identified if the point of convergence of afferents and the location of the primarily active motoneurons were described.

Central Afferent Systems

The convergent afferent systems include the maxillary branch of the fifth cranial nerve, and the ninth and tenth cranial nerves. These lead to the descending or spinal trigeminal system and the fasciculus and nucleus solitarius. The ninth and tenth cranial nerves admix considerably in terms of source and modality. It is thought provisionally that the parvicellular portion of nucleus solitarius is unlikely to constitute the afferent mechanism for swallowing. The nodose ganglion contains cells supplying sensory fibers to the abdominal and thoracic viscera rather than those having more relevance for swallowing. The magnocellular part of nucleus solitarius receives input from the cortex and the ventrolateral thalamus. Some fibers of the ninth and tenth cranial nerves project to the lateral cuneate nucleus (lateral portion of posterior spinal column), serving as a possible relay to the cerebellum. Clinical disorders such as palatomyoclonus may involve the inferior olive. Therefore, it appears to have an as yet unspecified special relationship to the pharyngeal and laryngeal musculature.

Motoneuron Pools

The motoneurons of interest in the neuroregulation of swallowing include the salivatory nuclei on either side of the genu of the seventh cranial nerve and the dorsal motor nucleus of the tenth cranial nerve, which may innervate the esophageal smooth muscle in man. Experiments to date have been ambiguous, since sectioning of the tenth cranial nerve distal to the recurrent laryngeal branch produces degeneration in the nucleus ambiguus as well as in the dorsal motor nucleus. Many neurons in the nucleus of the twelfth cranial nerve participate in swallowing. Histologic studies in patients with bulbar poliomyelitis revealed loss of neurons in rostral nucleus ambiguus in those who had dysphagia, whereas those with dysarthria were found to have cell loss in the caudal portions (Baker, Matzke, and Brown, 1950). These effects would be explained by representation of palatopharyngeal and esophageal musculature in the magnocellular part of the nucleus. Comparative studies have revealed great flexibility of human palatopharyngeal and laryngeal manipulation, reflecting progressive refinement of the controlling interneuronal network and the control exerted by the medullary reticular formation. Homologies exist in terms of the proprioceptive, monosynaptic pericellular structures surrounding motoneurons that have to do with deglutition, and those of the seventh cranial nerve, including the trajectory of existing axons.

Central Efferent Systems

The reflexes produced as a result of the afferent, central, and efferent systems currently under discussion have been divided into simple, direct, or "elementary" reflexes as opposed to more protracted and extensive sequences that culminate in normal swallowing. The elementary reflexes involve muscles responding to stimulation of the nasal mucosa, nasopharynx, and pharynx, and involve the following nerves: fifth, tenth, and eleventh cranial, lingual, and the SLN and recurrent laryngeal. As previously mentioned, the neuronal activities resulting in swallowing also overlap with those responsible for phonation, coughing, and speech. Normal swallowing appears to involve not only reflex initiation by way of several types of peripheral excitation, but a central facilitation of the swallowing center or its afferent pathways.

Experimental destruction of the center on one side of the medulla eliminates swallowing in the ipsilateral musculature except for the crossed constrictor pathway previously described. The responsiveness of the contralateral center to afferent input for the side of the lesion is still normal, however. For example, destruction of the left swallowing center does not prevent right-sided swallowing if the left SLN is stimulated. This has immediate clinical relevance, especially in the case of destructive lesions to the brainstem on one side. As previously outlined, voluntary efforts in the absence of reflex initiation from peripheral stimuli will not result in swallowing. The peripheral stimuli include water, light touch, and chemical stimulation. If we were to seek a principal point from which swallowing is most likely to be initiated, it would normally lie in the palatal area innervated by the maxillary branch of the fifth cranial nerve, although this may vary among species. For example, in cat and dog the principal effective area is the upper pharynx, innervated by the ninth cranial nerve.

The frontal motor cortex (lateral precentral gyrus) in primates and many other species produces a combination of chewing and swallowing movements with effects upon many structures of the neck, palate, tongue, and pharynx. These are usually bilateral. It appears that the swallowing elicited by direct cortical stimulation, and not by evoked or pharyngeal movement, follows a path through the ventral limb of the internal capsule that is largely extra-pyramidal. It is interesting that the type of reflex response (for example, swallowing versus gagging) depends on the spatiotemporal pattern of afferent action, even though the same set of pharyngeal or palatoreceptors is excited. This pluripotential nature of afferent activity is a hallmark of the complex neural organization under discussion, with special emphasis on the linkage between swallowing and respiration.

NEUROREGULATION OF THE GASTROESOPHAGEAL JUNCTION

The gastroesophageal junction is controlled largely by smooth muscle and is thus inhibited and relaxed by activity in afferent nerve fibers. This contrasts with the activity at the pharyngoesophageal junction where contraction evoked in striated muscle is relaxed by inhibition in the central nervous system (CNS). Inhibition of the gastroesophageal junction and esophagus proper is separable, but appears to depend upon the dorsal motor nucleus of the tenth cranial nerve, assuming it innervates the smooth muscle of the esophagus and stomach. Esophageal peristalsis may occur in the absence of buccopharyngeal swallowing, but is inhibited during activity of the swallowing center; another observation supporting the fact that swallowing is preceded by inhibition. Once the esophageal component has been initiated, further swallowing or stimulation of the ninth cranial nerve cannot alter completion of its course of action. The pattern of esophageal excitation is subject to feedback control. This is emphatically distinguished from the buccopharyngeal phase where feedback control is not apparent in the unchangeable course of events following the initiation of swallowing.

SUMMARY

A functional swallowing center appears to exist having selective mechanisms for activation by appropriate stimuli. These have a defined spatiotemporal code, with interconnection of component cells resulting in a virtually invariable sequence of excitation and inhibition so that swallowing is the same, regardless of its manner of initiation and with precision of organization resulting in control over relevant motoneurons. Corollaries of these features are that feedback regulation is not necessary for swallowing to proceed, that the output of the center is highly stable, and that activity in the center exerts inhibition upon possibly competing centers. The specific motoneuron pools involved in swallowing appear independent of the action of others in terms of the pattern of response. A clinical correlation was reported in a patient with severe bulbar poliomyelitis in whom the esophageal phase of swallowing was normal even though pharyngeal paralysis made it impossible to pass material from the mouth into the esophagus (Sanchez, Kramer, and Ingelfinger, 1953). If we conceive of the two half-centers of the total swallowing center functioning independently, then the concept of unilateral swallowing would involve pathways conveying constrictor excitation from one half-center probably to the contralateral nucleus ambiguus with decussation behind the obex. A single half-center appears to exert initial inhibition ipsilaterally and subsequent contralateral excitation by way of motoneurons to the lower constrictors. Intercenter coordination is extensive, with the possibility of connections between half-centers achieving mutual inhibition.

The swallowing center as defined by numerous studies reveals its location to be in the reticular substance between the posterior pole of the seventh nucleus and the anterior pole of the inferior olive. It is of clinical relevance that unilateral destruction in this area abolishes swallowing unilaterally, whereas partial destruction results in peculiar "fractionations" of swallowing activity (Doty, Richmond, and Storey, 1967); these have not been fully described from a clinical standpoint. Possibly, subcenters exist compromising the total half-center for swallowing on each side of the midline. It may be useful for the reader to study Figure 1.11, as it translates the neurologic process into graphic form.

REFERENCES

Ardran GM, Kemp FH. The mechanism of swallowing. Proc R Soc Med 1951;44:1038–40.

Ardran GM, Kemp FH. Protection of laryngeal airway during swallowing. Br J Radiol 1952;25:406–16.

Baker AB, Matzke HA, Brown JR. Poliomyelitis; bulbar poliomyelitis; a study of medullary function. Arch Neurol Psychiatry 1950;63:257–81.

Brown, Scott. Diseases of the ear, nose, and throat: the throat. Ballantyne J., and Groves J. eds. London: Butterworths, 1971.

Castell DO. Esophageal manometric studies: a perspective of their physiological and clinical relevance. J Clin Gastroenterol 1980;2:191–96.

Dodds WJ. Instrumentation and methods for intraluminal esophageal manometry. Arch Intern Med 1976;136:515–23.

Donner MW. Swallowing mechanisms and neuromuscular disorders. Semin Roentgenol 1974;9:273–82.

Donner M, Siegel C. The evaluation of neuromuscular disorders by cinefluorography. Am J Roentgenol 1965;94:299–307.

Doty RW, Bosma JF. Electromyographic analysis of reflex deglutition. J Neurophysiol 1956;19:44–60.

Doty RW, Richmond WH, Storey AT. Effect of medullary lesions on coordination of deglutition. Exp Neurol 1967;17:91–106.

Kaplan HM. Anatomy and physiology of speech: McGraw-Hill Series in Speech. New York: McGraw-Hill, 1960.

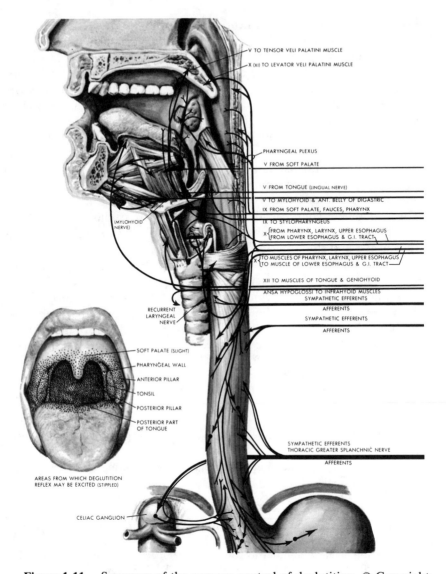

Figure 1.11. Summary of the nervous control of deglutition. © Copyright 1959, CIBA Pharmaceutical Company, Division of CIBA-GEIGY Corporation. Reprinted with permission, from THE CIBA COLLECTION OF MEDICAL ILLUSTRATIONS, illustrated by Frank H. Netter, M.D. All rights reserved.

Palmer ED. Disorders of the cricopharyngeus muscle: a review. Gastroenterology 1976;71:510–19.

Rontal M, Rontal E. Lesions of the vagus nerve: diagnosis, treatment, and rehabilitation. Laryngoscope 1977;87:72–86.

Sanchez GC, Kramer P, Ingelfinger FJ. Motor mechanisms of the esophagus, particularly its distal portion. Gastroenterology 1953;25:321–32.

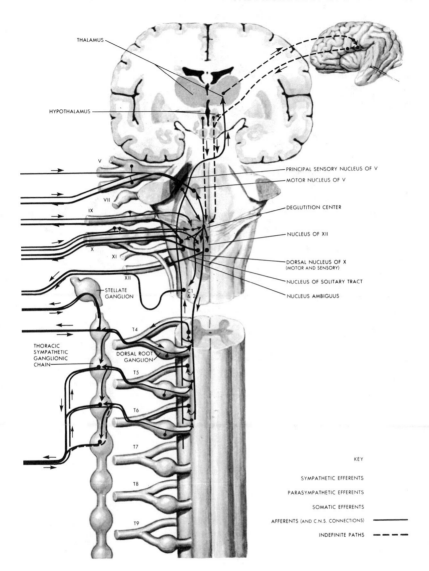

Figure 1.11. *(continued)*

Sasaki C. Paralysis of the larynx and pharynx. Surg Clin North Am 1980;60:1079–82.

Schultz A, Niemtzow P, Jacobs S, Naso F. Dysphagia associated with cricopharyngeal dysfunction. Arch Phys Med Rehabil 1979;60:381–6.

Sloan RF, Brummet SW, Westover JL, Ricketts RM, Ashley FL. Recent cinefluorographic advances in palatopharyngeal roentgenography. Am J Roentgenol 1964;92:977–85.

CHAPTER 2

Neurologic Disorders
of Swallowing
Roger M. Morrell

Discussion of the neurologic disorders of swallowing is preceded by some general remarks pertaining to the anatomic regions involved in the swallowing process as described in Chapter 1, and also with regard to the regional and hierarchical arrangement of levels within the nervous system. From the standpoint of the swallowing process itself, the considerations involve the progression from the oral cavity to the distal esophagus and stomach. From the standpoint of the nervous system, the major disorders are divided primarily into those that affect the smooth or striated musculature (myogenic) and those that affect central nervous system (CNS) centers, including the spinal cord and/or peripheral nerves (neurogenic). Finally, consideration is given to the major psychogenic disorders of swallowing.

GENERAL CONSIDERATIONS

The intimate relationship of the last four cranial nerves (ninth through twelfth) results in the possibility of many combinations of nerve lesions that have similar common pathways in terms of symptomatology. Examples include loss of strength of the voice, hoarseness, nasal speech, difficulty in swallowing, and nasal regurgitation or aspiration. Referred or directly mediated painful sensations in the region of the external ear and scalp may draw attention to the ninth and tenth cranial nerves, while weakness and wasting of the sternomastoids, trapezii, and tongue may implicate the eleventh and twelfth cranial nerves.

A neurologic cause of dysphagia is more likely if the anatomy is normal without deformity, although symmetry may be misleading since it may represent bilateral lesions. Deformity may occur in the presence of a sensory deficit, while asymmetry may result from a unilateral problem. Since the larynx is innervated by the tenth cranial nerve, paralysis of one or both vocal cords may be completely separate from neurologic involvement of the palatopharyngeal apparatus. Neurologic involvement of the orobuccal phase of swallowing is related to its volitional nature. Involvement of the reflexly controlled pharynx and the mixed functions of the larynx affect not only swallowing, but speaking and breathing, so that it is important to note associated functions. The symptoms associated with these functions (dysarthria, dysphagia, and dysphonia) may all coexist, as in parkinsonism or other disorders of the basal ganglia. It is difficult to attempt to determine the most likely neurologic localization from symptoms and signs affecting a highly coordinated process such as swallowing. This is apparent when we consider that not only basal ganglia but cerebellum and sensory feedback control are required to coordinate the voluntary as well as reflex muscle movements that permit precise manipulation of the bolus in a normal swallow.

Pathology of the brainstem affecting swallowing frequently takes the form of bulbar palsy, poliomyelitis, trauma, vascular abnormalities such as the Wallenberg's syndrome of the posterior inferior cerebellar artery, and brainstem tumors. The brainstem may also be involved in many congenital degenerative disorders, including hereditary spastic paralysis, familial dysautonomia, amyotrophic lateral sclerosis (ALS), and syringobulbia. A key finding associated with brainstem involvement is failure of the cricopharyngeus muscle to relax during swallowing, with accompanying pharyngeal retention, stasis, and nasal regurgitation (Schultz et al., 1979). As one-half of the brain activates the brainstem nuclei bilaterally, there would be no advantage in having the individual sides of the mouth and throat working separately. Therefore unilateral cerebral lesions often spare the brainstem.

It has been found that lesions of various levels of the CNS, particularly cerebellar, upper motoneuron, lower motoneuron, and extrapyramidal (parkinson-like), produce different and identifiable patterns of lingual, labial, and velar movement as examined cineradiographically (Logemann et al., 1977).

From a diagnostic standpoint, neurologic causes of swallowing disorders are generally identified through such factors as the duration of the swallowing process, difficulties with liquids and solids, nasal regurgitation, and the presence or absence of heartburn. Hoarseness may indicate intrinsic laryngeal disease or relate to carcinoma. It may be accompanied by recurrent laryngeal nerve paralysis complicating such diseases as polymyositis and dermatomyositis (Metheny, 1978). Bilateral nuclear involvement of the tenth cranial nerve may be present in both poliomyelitis and polyneuritis. A prominent symptom of dysarthria may be present in ALS, while coughing, especially as a function of the recumbent position, may relate to Zenker's diverticulum, achalasia, or esophageal-tracheal fistula. Hiccup suggests phrenic or diaphragmatic involvement and sometimes accompanies carcinoma and achalasia.

This chapter does not detail the elements of physical examination as it relates to neurologic disorders of swallowing, although certain physical and neurologic signs are reviewed in appropriate sections. It is of interest to itemize conditions related to hypocontractility or lack of contractility of the peripheral region. In this connection, pharyngeal striated muscle may be hypocontractile in the case of poly (dermato) myositis, myasthenia gravis, myotonic dystrophy, diabetic neuropathy, and amyloidosis. Furthermore, syndromes overlap, such as collagen or connective tissue disease and progressive systemic sclerosis, systemic lupus erythematosus (SLE) and polyarteritis nodosa, and progressive systemic sclerosis and SLE. Esophageal smooth muscle may be hypocontractile in scleroderma or progressive systemic sclerosis, in lupus erythematosus, rheumatoid arthritis, periarteritis nodosa, Raynaud's syndrome, diabetic neuropathy, alcoholic neuropathy, and myxedema.

In regional peripheral evaluation, oropharyngeal dysphagia is accompanied by a decreased gag reflex, weakness of cervical or facial muscles, and often a speech disorder. It is a common cause of dysphagia, and if it progresses to pharyngeal paralysis, it may include a number of sensory changes secondary to painful lesions of the mouth or tongue. Such diseases include scarlet fever, mumps, viral infections, herpes, monilia, peritonsilar abscess, carcinoma, or syphilis. Acute thyroiditis also may be a cause. Pharyngeal paralysis eventually often results from poliomyelitis, syringomyelia, multiple sclerosis, cerebrovascular accident involving the brainstem, and diphtheritic neuritis of the ninth and tenth cranial nerves. Muscle weakness leading to pharyngeal involvement is found in myasthenia gravis, myotonic dystrophies, amyloidosis, scleroderma, and dermatomyositis. Other conditions to be considered in the oropharyngeal phase are Plummer-Vinson syndrome, laryngeal fixations secondary to carcinoma, tuberculosis or syphilis, and congenital abnormalities of the tongue and palate. Plummer-Vinson syndrome includes dysphagia, glossitis, hypochromic anemia, and sometimes splenomegaly and achlorhydria (absence of free hydrochloric acid in the stomach). It is often thought to have a dysphagic component that may be due in part to psychic or emotional (hysteria-like) achalasia of the cricopharyngeus muscle. Pharyngeal involvement in such syndromes and others previously mentioned relates to inability of pharyngeal constrictors to initiate peristaltic contraction and empty contents of the pharynx into the esophagus. An isolated pharyngeal palsy may be difficult to evaluate and may result from selective involvement of the nerve supply from the superior branches of the vagus emanating from the cephalic region of the nucleus ambiguus where pharyngeal function is bilateral in terms of motor cortical activity (O'Connor, 1976). Furthermore, it has been pointed out in Chapter 1 that lesions of the vagus nerve may produce devastating effects on the functions of swallowing, breathing, and phonation. Sasaki (1980) discussed this in terms of low vagal paralysis (below the nodose ganglion) that rarely affects deglutition, and high vagal paralysis (above the nodose ganglion), which is catastrophic whether unilateral or bilateral. The difference may lie, in part, with the fact that the higher paralysis often is accompanied by widespread involvement of the fifth, seventh, ninth, and twelfth cranial nerves with the overriding threat of aspiration. Most neurologic causes of oropharyngeal dysphagia are chronic or intermittent and need to be analyzed in terms of the foregoing considerations.

Specific causes of laryngeal involvement in the peripheral arrangement of swallowing include herpes zoster (Pahor, 1979), mitral valve disease causing paralysis of the left vocal fold and dysphagia (Morgan and Mourant, 1980), and intrinsic pathologies such as Crohn's disease with granulomatous changes of larynx and pharynx. Secondary amyloidosis also may produce dysphagia. Since the principal function of the larynx is sphincteric, interruption of reflexes responsible for laryngeal closure result in failure to elevate and close the larynx by contraction of intrinsic laryngeal adductor musculature by way of the sensory limbs of the ninth and tenth cranial nerves. Failure of these mechanisms on a neurologic basis also may include failure to inhibit respiration reflexly or to open the larynx appropriately during inspiration by contraction of the laryngeal abductors. As a result, neurologic disease of the larynx may cause not only aspiration, but stridor and air hunger.

MYOGENIC DISORDERS OF SWALLOWING

Myopathies and Myotonias

For purposes of this discussion, myopathies and myotonias include the dystrophies (i.e., Duchenne's disease) and conditions such as dermatomyositis or polymyositis, which may be harbingers of systemic carcinoma or disease entities in their own right, as listed below:

1. Myopathies and myotonias, dystrophies
2. Dermatomyositis or polymyositis
3. Dysthyroid conditions
4. Myasthenia gravis
5. Neuromuscular esophageal disorders
   a. Scleroderma
   b. Raynaud's disease
   c. Achalasia
   d. Diffuse spasm

The dysphagia and dysphonia of myotonic dystrophy often are accompanied by the pathognomonic features of bilateral facial weakness, temporal balding, cataracts, and extensive peripheral and palatal weakness. Myotonia of the tongue usually is demonstrated by placing a tongue blade flat beneath the tongue and another on edge above the midportion of the tongue. A subsequent impact causes a constrictive band across the top of the tongue. The myopathy of dermatomyositis, acute systemic lupus erythematosus, or oculopharyngeal myopathy involves degenerative or inflammatory changes seen pathologically in muscle. It is demonstrated radiographically by abnormal deglutition, particularly prolongation of muscular activity and weakened or shallow pharyngeal contractions, with retention in pharyngeal recesses with stasis. In myotonia dystrophica, pharyngeal swallow may be only slightly impaired with restricted contraction, or result in complete paralysis leading to nasal and tracheal aspiration. Successive swallows frequently show both improvement in pharyngeal contraction and decreased duration.

Myopathies often are congenital. They usually eventually involve symmetric proximal weakness with patterned wasting depending on the type of myopathy; absence of sensory symptomatology; abnormal electromyography, muscle biopsy, and electrocardiogram; and occasionally, diagnostic patterns of muscle enzyme abnormalities. As an autosomal dominant disorder, myotonic dystrophy may involve the pharynx and esophagus with resultant dysphagia, nasal regurgitation, and aspiration of ingested fluid (Harvey, Sherbourne, and Siegel, 1965). Symptoms apparently result from abnormal esophageal peristalsis, pooling in the pharynx, inability to propel a normal bolus into the upper esophagus, prominent failure to initiate swallowing of water, and prolongation of contraction and relaxation phases in both upper and lower esophagus. An atonic dilated esophagus may be an additional feature. Aspiration of pharyngeal contents into the larynx and bronchial tree with possible bronchiectasis has been associated with myotonic dystrophy (Ludman 1962). Pierce, Creamer, and MacDermott (1965) described consistent esophageal peristaltic abnormalities in myotonic dystrophy.

Another myogenic disorder known as oculopharyngeal dystrophy is a chronic progressive external ophthalmoplegia occurring in older age groups and characterized by ptosis and dysphagia in an autosomal dominant pattern first described in French-Canadian families. It must be distinguished from such ocular conditions as Graefe's disease, descending ocular myopathy, ophthalmoplegia plus (with retinal pigmentary anomalies, cardiac disorders, etc.), and other heredoataxias. Various *formes frustes* (atypical forms) also complicate the diagnosis, as outlined in the review by Bastiaensen and Schulte (1979). Typically, there are reduced or absent pharyngeal reflexes and weak movements of the soft palate, tongue, and larynx. Cineradiography reveals stagnation in the pyriform sinuses, paresis of pharyngeal muscles, and abnormal relaxation of the cricopharyngeal sphincter. The most important cause of dysphagia is absence of reflex relaxation, which requires a rise in pressure in the lower part of the pharynx. Dysphagia results when this pressure rise does not occur due to pharyngeal muscular dystrophy. Diagnosis depends on the involvement of other cranial muscles, myopathic facies, and electromyographic findings characteristic of myopathy. Some patients have increased levels of creatinine phosphokinase (CPK, a blood enzyme) or abnormal immunoglobulins. The disorder must be distinguished from myasthenia gravis and progressive bulbar paralysis; myotonic dystrophy; polymyositis; tumors; inflammation of the brainstem, meninges, and skull base; senile changes with or without organic stenosis of the esophagus; syphilis;

and the other ocular dystrophic conditions as mentioned. Bosch, Gowans, and Munsat (1979) described a patient with secondary inflammatory changes of muscle similar to those of idiopathic polymyositis. Duranceau and associates (1978) drew attention in oculopharyngeal dystrophy to prominent oropharyngeal dysphagia secondary to pharyngo-oral and pharyngonasal regurgitation associated with chronic aspiration and bronchorrhea.

Diagnosis of dysthyroid conditions depends on generalized weakness and reflex abnormality. Often, the examiner finds a pendular quality to reflexes in a setting of documented abnormality of thyroid metabolism based on quantitative hormone determination and, to some extent, response to therapy.

Myasthenia Gravis

Myasthenia gravis is a disorder that should be considered in any healthy adult with laryngeal weakness, varying dysphonia, and dysphagia (Figure 2.1). These manifestations may respond dramatically to a diagnostic injection of intravenous edrophonium (Tensilon). Not all patients with bulbar myasthenia exhibit ptosis or diplopia, which may be commonly associated with the pharyngeal involvement seen more often in younger patients. Indirect laryngoscopy is indicated, together with fluoroscopic studies of deglutition. Symptoms of myasthenia gravis are similar to those of ordinary fatigue and many psychologic disturbances, especially if pharyngeal or laryngeal involvement is not accompanied by other neurologic signs. Motoneuron disease (ALS) also should be considered in the differential diagnosis, given clinical manifestations of progressive dysarthria, dysphagia, and dysphonia occurring in otherwise healthy patients over 30 years of age.

Myasthenia gravis causes impaired conduction at the myoneural junction of striated muscles. Dysphagia is an early sign and is accompanied by ocular muscle fatigue. Swallowing worsens late in the day and at the end of each meal, but is not accompanied by spasm or hypertrophy of the cricopharyngeal sphincter, a feature that may be seen in brainstem lesions, sideropenic (iron-deficiency) dysphagia, or pharyngoesophageal incoordination. Dysphagia may occur during treatment of myasthenia gravis, due to either cholinergic crisis resulting from relative overdose of anticholinesterases or less commonly, aggressive steroid therapy.

Carpenter, McDonald, and Howard (1979) reported that 30 percent of 175 myasthenic patients had oral, pharyngeal, or laryngeal complaints. One-half of the 30 percent had dysphagia, 13 percent dysarthria, and 2 percent had dysphonia. The prominence of these symptoms and signs may give rise to an erroneous diagnosis of primary bulbar involvement. Eaton and Lambert (1957) described a myasthenic syndrome associated with malignant tumors that caused proximal limb weakness and prominent cranial nerve symptom-

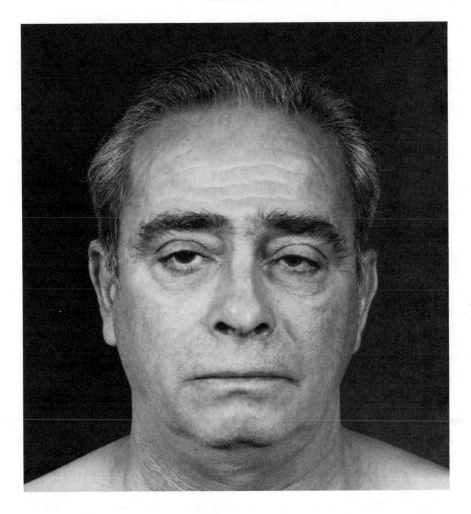

Figure 2.1. Patient with myasthenia gravis demonstrating ocular muscle fatigue. Note ptosis of both eyelids. This patient also had marked facial and tongue weakness, dysphagia, and dysphonia.

atology, including dry mouth and in some cases reports of impotence. Some patients appear to manifest a cholinergic dysautonomia (Rubenstein, Horowitz, and Bender, 1979). Botulinum intoxication and Sjögren's syndrome are in the differential diagnosis. Although space does not permit a detailed account of the pathophysiology of Eaton-Lambert syndrome, it is due to a defect of acetylcholine release from presynaptic terminals, rather than the highly specific autoimmune receptor defect to which myasthenia gravis is attributed.

Traumatic Myositis

Metheny (1978) has described the vocal and swallowing disorders associated with traumatic myositis. Often present are dysphagia, dysphonia, and weakness of the tongue with radiologic "gaping" or vallecular sign, and defective propulsion of the bolus with altered esophageal motility. This disorder must be differentiated from disseminated lupus erythematosus and scleroderma. Although it is a rare collagen or connective tissue disorder, there is a 50 percent mortality rate within the first two years which may relate to its association with primary carcinoma. There is striking creatinuria, dermatitis, periorbital heliotrope, edema, and proximal symmetrical muscle weakness. Electromyographic and biopsy results are supportive of the diagnosis, with electromyography guiding the area to be biopsied.

Neuromuscular Disorders of the Esophagus

Some general principles may assist in elucidating the problem areas and clinical entities associated with neuromuscular esophageal disorders.

Conditions leading to esophageal dysphagia may affect the upper esophageal sphincter (cricopharyngeal portion) or the lower esophageal sphincter. It may be accompanied by sticking sensations, need to drink liquids to push the bolus, and disproportionate problems with solid foods. In patients in the lower age range (10 to 45 years), common causes include achalasia, scleroderma, constrictive ring, and spasm. Above age 45, carcinoma and peptic esophagitis are more frequent causes.

The scope of this chapter does not allow an exhaustive review of all neuromuscular causes of esophageal motility disorders. A useful review is provided by Fischer and associates (1965). They described 42 patients who were divided into broad categories of cerebrovascular disease, Parkinson's disease, ALS, multiple sclerosis (MS), peripheral neuropathy, undiagnosed central nervous system disease, myasthenia gravis, thyrotoxic myopathy, and myotonic dystrophy. The most striking abnormalities were primarily in myopathic disorders such as myasthenia gravis and myotonic dystrophy. Decrease in peristaltic waves with or without spasm could be found in patients with lesions in many locations, central or peripheral. Additionally, patients with ALS exhibited impaired upper sphincter activity. Those with pseudobulbar palsy and Parkinson's disease exhibited decreased peristalsis.

Abnormalities of motility appear to be associated anatomically with vagal involvement at the supranuclear, nuclear, or peripheral levels. Pharyngeal dysphagia may result from disorders associated with nonperistaltic episodes including segmental spasm. These disorders have come to be called high dysphagia. Although our emphasis in this chapter is on neurologic disease, it must be mentioned, especially in connection with the lower esophageal sphincter, that neuropharmacologic effects may be significant. Cholinergic agonists and metoclopramide increase tone, whereas alcohol and anticholinergic substances decrease it.

Intrinsic Esophageal Disorders

A useful introduction to the problems of intrinsic esophageal muscular disorders or conditions of neuromuscular origin is the article by Vantrappen and co-workers (1979). Achalasia predominantly occurs in the third, fourth, and fifth decades. The esophagus is dilated with symptoms of obstruction, regurgitation, and possibly early pain. Achalasia is due to motor failure and is characterized by feeble and incoordinated contractions. It must be distinguished from diffuse spasm, which is less common, usually occurs after age 60 years, is generally accompanied by significant substernal pain during swallowing, and exhibits diffuse spastic narrowing on radiography, with segmental constriction or pseudodiverticulum formation. Simultaneous and repetitive contractions of considerable amplitude occur in the smooth muscle of the esophagus in contrast to the findings in achalasia. Manometry may be necessary to diagnose diffuse spasm. The term vigorous achalasia describes a condition that differs from either of the above by exhibiting simultaneous repetitive contractions after swallowing, but with decreased amplitude and more pain than with achalasia. Achalasia must be differentiated from megaesophagus or Chagas's disease (ganglionic cell fallout), and from cardiospasm or functional obstruction of the esophagus at the level of the hiatus with thoracic esophageal dilatation. Enlargement of the esophagus may occur in esophageal dyssynergia due to failed relaxation of the distal esophagus.

A generalized disease known as scleroderma or progressive systemic sclerosis may involve the esophagus, with abnormal manometric signs appearing before clinical symptoms are noted. Esophageal involvement is more prevalent in patients with associated Raynaud's disease (acrosclerosis: scleroderma of upper extremities). Again, neuromuscular failure of the smooth muscle portion of the esophagus exists with retention of peristalsis in the striated muscle.

It is important to recognize that neuromuscular disorders affecting the esophagus may exhibit similar manometric abnormalities, yet be widely different in terms of etiology or specificity. For example, abnormal manometric patterns with decreased motility or absent peristalsis may be found in myasthenia gravis, myotonic dystrophy, the peripheral neuropathy of diabetes or alcoholism, and Parkinson's disease; whereas MS may reveal changes characteristic of diffuse spasm, which also may occur as a result of cerebrovascular accidents. A fallacious terminology has crept into the literature with the appearance of the term "bulbar palsy" describing abnormal relaxation of the upper esophageal sphincter resulting from pharyngoesophageal involvement. This term should be reserved for conditions that result from pathology affecting the brainstem, its nuclei, and peripheral cranial nerves or their respective branches. Myotonic dystrophy and myasthenia gravis, therefore, are not bulbar palsies, even though the muscles affected are those innervated by the brainstem.

Students of esophageal disorders have subdivided diffuse spasm and achalasia into phases or stages with reference to variations in segmental esophageal differences in neuromuscular tone. Pope (1977) drew attention to the difficulty of classifying esophageal disorders. He stated that diffuse spasm is more rare and may be more difficult to classify. Although myotomies of various kinds have been promoted for the treatment of spasm in numerous segments of the esophagus, their efficacy has not been widely documented by manometric or cineradiographic studies. Latimer (1981) reported the effective use of biofeedback and self-regulation in the treatment of one case of diffuse spasm. Diffuse spasm was reported by Peppercorn, Docken, and Rosenberg (1979) in association with systemic lupus erythematosus. The concept of presbyesophagus has met some resistance in view of the fact that many elderly individuals have decreased amplitude of esophageal propulsive contractions; however, symptomatic disorders of motility or dysphagia imply disease and require specific evaluation and diagnosis.

NEUROGENIC DISORDERS OF SWALLOWING

The principal neurogenic causes of dysphagia are as follows:

1. Riley-Day syndrome
2. Acquired central disorders
    a. Stroke syndromes and vascular disorders
        (1) Capsular infarct
        (2) Lacunar disease
        (3) Pseudobulbar palsy
        (4) Apraxias and agnosias
        (5) Brainstem stroke
        (6) Vasculitis
    b. Movement disorders
        (1) Parkinson's disease
        (2) Dystonias and dyskinesias
        (3) Huntington's disease
        (4) Palatal myoclonus
    c. Poliomyelitis and other systemic infections
        (1) Diphtheria
        (2) Botulism
        (3) Rabies
        (4) Tetanus
    d   Amyotrophic lateral sclerosis

e. Other causes
    (1) Dementias
    (2) Multiple sclerosis
    (3) Tuberculosis
    (4) Syphilis
    (5) Neoplasms
    (6) Degenerative disorders
3. Acquired peripheral disorders
    a. Recurrent laryngeal neuropathy
    b. Cranial neuropathies
        (1) Diabetes
        (2) Leukemia
        (3) Lymphoma
        (4) Carcinoma
    c. Other neuropathies
4. Neurodevelopmental disorders
    a. Syringomyelia and syringobulbia
    b. Klippel-Feil syndrome
    c. Arnold-Chiari syndrome
    d. Cerebral palsy
    e. Other

Riley-Day Syndrome

Riley-Day syndrome is a congenital and familial dysautonomia of autorecessive genetic pattern that includes feeding problems associated with dysphagia. It is accompanied by different degrees of sensory neuropathy that involve afferent impulses.

Stroke Syndromes

Stroke syndromes are numerous and can be confusing in terms of their effects on swallowing, depending upon whether the predominant features of the syndrome are upper or lower motoneuronal.

Upper Motoneuron Syndromes

The upper motoneuron syndromes include diseases of the cortex, internal capsule, and suprabulbar areas adjacent to the hypothalamus, as well as posterior and descending tracts within the internal capsule beneath the genu. These lesions, regardless of size, may affect both voluntary corticospinal pathways and reflex connections by means of partial or complete interruption of corticobulbar pathways. Bilateral lesions are always more severe since there is bilateral representation in the brainstem, which may be spared functionally by a unilateral hemispheral lesion. Infarctions of the internal capsule often involve hemisensory deficits as well as hemianopia (visual field defect).

Lacunar disease eventually may be related to multi-infarct dementia and is usually associated with hypertension. There are no specific or diagnostic swallowing defects associated with these clinically defined entities. Pseudobulbar palsy is due to suprasegmental interruption of cortical influences on the lower bulbar musculature with resultant functional disruption. Bilateral cortical bulbar interruption results in dysarthric speech, dysphagia, drooling, strangling on attempt at drinking, impaired gag reflex, and susceptibility to aspiration. Interpersonal contact or stimulus may sometimes result in laughing or crying without appropriately associated emotional content. Frontal release reflexes such as grasp, snout, or suck may occur as a result of bilateral cerebral infarctions leading to this syndrome. Also, ALS and advanced MS may cause this disorder.

Apraxias and agnosias may result from stroke that affects higher cortical function at the cognitive level. They interfere with coordination of a voluntary movement or a series of movements based on a disconnection between the neural processing required to elaborate it and the motor sequence required to carry it out. Apraxias and agnosias often accompany aphasia with its characteristic cognitive abnormalities of language and thinking. The neuromuscular apparatus for swallowing may be normal, yet the motor concept is not transmitted in a sequential fashion. "Swallowing agnosia" has not been described, but should be acknowledged as a possibility on theoretical grounds.

Brainstem Stroke

Strokes affecting the brainstem are becoming more common and are extremely important, but may be confusing to the non-neurologist because of the number of eponymic descriptions associated with them. The vascular supply to the brainstem can be considered to be divided into two major subdivisions: the medial one-third and the lateral two-thirds. Vascular occlusions or ischemia occurring in either region will affect the structures within that region, and the resulting functional abnormalities reflect the ischemic deficits of the deprived tissue. Strokes of the brainstem that affect structures involved in the control of swallowing usually affect the cricopharyngeal muscle's ability to relax. Again, we note that one-half of the brain activates brainstem nuclei bilaterally, and therefore unilateral brain lesions spare the brainstem. Some brainstem strokes, however, especially hemorrhages, may cross the midline in the region of the pons, affecting a volume of tissue in the rostrocaudal dimension aside from anatomic partial transection of the brainstem.

A classic brainstem vascular syndrome affecting swallowing is that of Wallenberg; it is secondary to occlusion of a dominant vertebral artery or the posterior inferior cerebral artery, a branch of the vertebral. Typically, the patient has vertigo, nausea, vomiting, prostration with severe ataxia followed by hiccups, nystagmus and gaze abnormalities, and few sensory complaints. Clinical examination reveals an absent ipsilateral corneal reflex and analgesia of the ipsilateral upper face accompanied by ipsilateral Horner's syndrome. There is hoarseness due to paralysis of the ipsilateral vocal fold (incomplete) and paresis of the ipsilateral palate. Further examination reveals diminution of pain and temperature on the opposite side of the body. The ischemia or infarction affects the lateral medulla and vertigo results from involvement of the vestibular complex. Involvement of the descending nucleus and tract of the fifth cranial nerve causes the corneal and facial analgesia, while crossed thermal loss is caused by involvement of the spinothalamic tract and nucleus of the fifth cranial nerve carrying pain and temperature from the opposite side of the body. Examination of a cross-sectional diagram of the medulla reveals that ischemia of the lateral two-thirds produces ipsilateral ataxia due to involvement of the restiform body (Figure 2.2). Palatal and laryngeal weakness, sometimes accompanied by hiccups, reflect involvement of the nucleus ambiguus and may require tracheostomy, although recovery is expected.

Strokes affecting the basilar artery may produce palatal myoclonus, a rhythmic jerking at frequencies of 80 to 120 beats per minute that also may include muscles of the face, neck, larynx, tongue, and eyes. This appears to involve the dentate nucleus of the cerebellum, red nucleus of the basal ganglia, and inferior olive of the brainstem, together with the central tegmental tract connecting the red nucleus and inferior olive in the tegmental pons. Infarction of the paramedian pons as a result of occlusive arterial disease is often signaled by internuclear ophthalmoplegia. This also may be a common finding in MS, but is not limited to it.

Most brainstem strokes that specifically involve structures underlying swallowing affect the medulla and possibly the vagal nuclei or peripheral nerves as they exit. The same brainstem structures that are affected by occlusive arterial disease may also be affected by irritative or inflammatory arterial disease in the form of vasculitis. Vasculitis may be associated with connective tissue disorders or may be idiopathic or immune-related. Just as the diagnosis of arterial occlusive disease depends upon associated risk factors and evidence of arterial disease on angiography, vasculitis occurs in a setting of immunologic abnormalities such as drug abuse, and may require a full angiographic investigation.

Movement Disorders

Of the movement disorders that consistently affect swallowing, Parkinson's disease is of special importance. It is a common neurologic disorder characterized by tremor and/or muscular rigidity, and/or bradykinesia or akinesia with dysarthric speech, a shuffling walk, and an expressionless stare or mask-like facies. It is caused by a deficiency of dopamine, which is produced by cells of the substantia nigra that affect basal ganglia function. Disorders of deglutition and esophageal function in Parkinson's disease are relatively

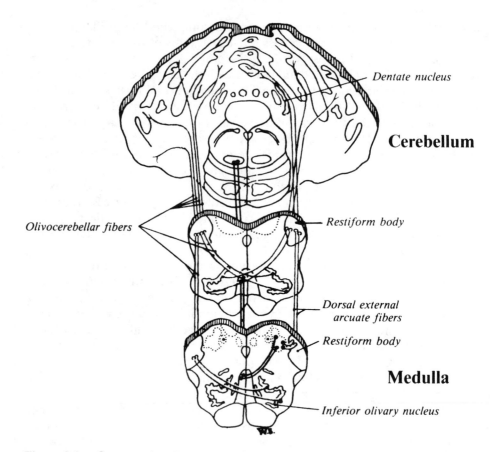

Figure 2.2.   Cross-sectional representation of medullar-cerebellar tracts illustrating how ischemic involvement of the lateral medulla can involve the restiform body and its cerebellar connections. Therefore, dysphagia resulting from brainstem stroke may also be accompanied by ataxia. Adapted and reprinted by permission of the publisher, from Everett, *Functional neuroanatomy,* Philadelphia: Lea & Febiger, 1967.

common (Pallis, 1971). This may include rapid weight loss with dysphagia, leading to a search for primary carcinoma. There may be delay in the initiation of swallow, irregular movement of the epiglottis, and stasis in the pyriform fossae and valleculae. Esophageal motility may be reduced, resulting in defects of peristalsis. Autonomic dysfunction may be partially responsible for the dysphagia, together with other autonomic signs, including sialorrhea (drooling), seborrhea, and orthostatic hypotension. Urinary incontinence may also be a feature. Some of these signs are related to pathologic changes in the dorsal vagal nucleus, sympathetic ganglia, locus ceruleus (floor of fourth ventricle), and hypothalamus. These have been summarized by Lieberman and colleagues (1980). The dysphagia has been described by

Calne and colleagues (1970), and specific abnormalities in esophageal motility by Bramble, Cunliffe, and Dellipiani (1978). Dystonias and dyskinesias (notably tardive dyskinesia) also may affect elements of deglutition, most commonly, the orobuccal phase. Huntington's disease is an example of a choreiform disorder that may affect the coordination of swallowing, especially in the late stages of disease.

Systemic Infections

Several infections or intoxications result in disorders of swallowing. Bulbar poliomyelitis may do so by direct involvement of neurons of the brainstem comprising the neural control of aspects of swallow described in Chapter 1. A diphtheritic polyneuropathy may affect the swallowing musculature in a completely separate manner from direct diphtheritic extension in the oropharynx. The toxin elaborated in botulism paralyzes the pharyngolaryngeal musculature. In rabies (rare in humans) there may be involvement of brainstem or medullary neurons similar to that of poliomyelitis secondary to the rabies virus. Dysphagia has been described as a primary symptom of tetanus (Weider and Tingwald, 1970).

Amyotrophic Lateral Sclerosis

Amyotrophic lateral sclerosis is a disease of insidious onset characterized by degeneration of motor units as a result of involvement of upper and lower motoneurons. It causes spastic and atrophic symptoms in the cranial, spinal, and peripheral musculature. It often affects the motoneurons of the brainstem, resulting in bulbar palsy with prominent slurred speech, hoarseness and breathiness, dysphagia, and dyspnea. The progressive deterioration of speech and swallow have been described by Dworkin and Hartman (1979). Since there is both spasticity and flaccidity as a result of upper and lower motoneuron involvement, there are effects on three levels of the upper airway: articulatory or speech-related, velopharyngeal (palatine pharynx), and phonatory (larynx).

Tongue weakness is apparent and the palate and larynx are affected by disorders in the ninth and tenth cranial nerves. These changes have been detailed by Carpenter, McDonald, and Howard (1978) and McGuirt and Blalock (1980). Management issues have been discussed by Delisa and associates (1979) and Smith and Norris (1975). As a result of pharyngeal dysphagia in ALS, there may be concomitant dilatation of the stomach and first part of the duodenum. Cineradiographic disorders of the pharynx in ALS have been described by Bosma and Brodie (1969), while pressure measurements have been detailed by Smith, Mulder, and Code (1957).

In concluding a brief account of acquired central nervous disorders, several diagnoses must be considered with respect to possible effects on deglutition. These include the dementias such as Alzheimer's disease, as well as MS, tuberculosis, syphilis, neoplasms of various types, and so-called degenerative disorders. Some of the neoplasms are of particular interest. For example, in addition to causing cerebellar signs of nausea, vertigo, and veering, certain cerebellar hemangioblastomas may produce hoarseness and strangling on fluids. The palatal weakness and vocal fold paresis are explained by so-called pressure palsies of cranial nerves that are more often associated with cerebellar masses than is commonly recognized. In considering intracranial mass or expanding lesions, abscess and syringobulbia must not be overlooked. The four lowest cranial nerves, especially the first three that exit from the same foramen, may be involved in several malignant diseases including nasopharyngeal carcinoma. From a diagnostic standpoint, neural involvement of swallowing mechanisms by neoplasms is usually progressive.

ACQUIRED PERIPHERAL DISORDERS

Cranial Nerve Neuropathies

The most important peripheral cranial neuropathy is secondary to involvement of the vagus (tenth cranial nerve) or its branches. Remembering that the fifth, seventh, ninth, tenth, and twelfth cranial nerves are involved in the neural control of swallowing, with inclusion of the eleventh for certain functions, it becomes apparent that pathology of one or more of these nerves may result in dysphagia. Specific involvement of these cranial nerves can occur as a result of several conditions that "normally" affect them. For example, a cerebellopontine angle tumor may compress the fifth and seventh cranial nerves, resulting in forms of dysfunction. The most common of these tumors are the acoustic neurinoma or meningioma with early symptoms of deafness, tinnitus, and facial numbness secondary to involvement of the fifth, seventh, and eighth cranial nerves. These may progress to direct compression or distortion of the brainstem, leading to pharyngeal and laryngeal symptomatology. Similarly, the seventh cranial nerve may be affected by Bell's palsy, and may be involved bilaterally, particularly in its motor branches. This is found in postinfectious myeloradiculopathies such as Guillain-Barré syndrome.

A prominent example of involvement of the tenth cranial nerve is paralysis of the vocal fold (usually left) and dysphagia occurring in the course of mitral valve disease (Morgan and Mourant, 1980). These may occur separately or in combination, and are thought to result from compression of the recurrent laryngeal nerve as it passes around the aortic arch. Dysphagia also may develop as a result of damage to autonomic nerve plexuses supplying the esophagus. This leads to abnormal peristalsis that may result from external compression by a tense left atrium. The ninth, tenth, eleventh, and twelfth cranial nerves are most commonly coinvolved in jugular venous bulb thrombosis, direct spread of nasopharyngeal carcinoma, or leukemic or lymphomatous infiltration along the base of the skull. The left recurrent laryngeal nerve may be damaged by carcinoma near the hilum of the left lung or by enlargement of several lymph nodes at that site. The right recurrent nerve may be affected by carcinoma at the lung apex or by tuberculosis and vascular abnormalities such as subclavian aneurysm. Although syphilitic aortitis is uncommon, this cardiovascular manifestation of tertiary syphilis may cause or be accompanied by dysphagia resulting from left recurrent laryngeal nerve involvement and connoted clinically by the well-known brassy cough. The nodose ganglion, located within the skull but outside the medulla, is the point of bifurcation of the main trunk of the vagus into the superior laryngeal nerve, which then subdivides peripherally into its motor and sensory branches (see Figures 1.8 and 1.9 [pages 25, 26] for anatomic reference). Catastrophic lesions above the nodose ganglion, even though external to the medulla, often result in bilateral total laryngeal paralysis with denervation of the pharynx. Lesions below the nodose ganglion usually are less life threatening, primarily because of diminished probability of aspiration.

Diabetic neuropathies usually only affect the oculomotor cranial nerves, although other cranial nerves may be damaged.

Infectious and peri-infectious involvement of cranial nerves occurs in herpes, diphtheria, and botulism, all of which may produce degrees of dysphonia and dysphagia that require early and drastic emergency measures. Since the conditions themselves may be self-limited, survival and/or reversibility of deficits often are dependent on appropriate and skillful management, particularly nursing care.

Amyloidosis (metabolic disorder marked by accumulation of amyloid deposits) may cause an autonomic neuropathy or directly infiltrate any of the cranial nerves, resulting in disordered deglutition.

Carter (1978) has reviewed postvagotomy dysphagia, and Pahor (1979) has reviewed herpes zoster of the larynx. The latter may accompany or be discrete from aural and facial herpes.

Cranial neuropathies secondary to leukemia, lymphoma, and carcinoma may evidence direct infiltration of cranial nerves with or without expansion and compression against unyielding bone, bony lesions with collapse of periforaminal conduits for cranial nerves, extraneural growth of infiltrating or metastasizing lesions, and enlarged lymphatic structures, or any combination of these disorders.

The cranial nerves may be affected by many disorders that rarely affect peripheral nerves and therefore even though they are peripheral to the central nervous system, they form a special category. Since numerous cranial nerves are involved at a particular site, they can be discussed in terms of site, those involved, usual pathologic cause, and eponymic syndrome.

At the cerebellopontine angle, in addition to involvement of the fifth and seventh cranial nerves, dysphagia may be secondary to possible disease of the ninth cranial nerve. At the jugular foramen, the ninth, tenth, and eleventh cranial nerves may be damaged by tumors or aneurysms (Vernet's syndrome); at the posterior laterocondylar space, cranial nerves nine through twelve, usually caused by tumors of parotid gland, carotid body, and secondary or metastatic tumors (Collet-Sicard syndrome); and at the posterior retroparotid space, cranial nerves nine through twelve with Horner's syndrome, caused by tumors of parotid, carotid body, and lymph node expansions including tuberculous adenitis (lymph gland inflammation). Although brainstem syndromes were previously discussed, it is often the case that certain cranial nerves are affected regularly, together with brainstem syndromes. Those of interest in relation to dysphagia or dysphagia/dysphonia include the following: (1) tegmentum of the medulla—involvement of the tenth cranial nerve, the corticospinal tract, with Horner's syndrome secondary to ischemic necrosis or tumor resulting in paralysis of soft palate, vocal fold, and a contralateral hemiplegia, or Avellis' syndrome; (2) tegmentum of the medulla—tenth and twelfth cranial nerves, corticospinal tract, Avellis' syndrome and ipsilateral tongue paralysis, soft palate and vocal fold paralysis, and contralateral hemiplegia, or Jackson's syndrome; and (3) Wallenberg's syndrome (previously described). The pathologies that may be encountered resulting in Wallenberg's syndrome include meningioma, cholesteatomas, and sarcomas, in addition to neurinoma and carcinoma. Chordomas may affect a succession of lower cranial nerves, giving rise to any of these syndromes. When a motor disorder does not cause atrophy, the question of myasthenia gravis must be raised.

Other Acquired Peripheral Disorders

Other acquired peripheral disorders affecting cranial nerves include neuropathies such as glossopharyngeal neuritis (etiology unknown, possibly analogous to Bell's palsy), and ankylosing vertebral hyperostosis (Leclercq and DeRobbio, 1978). The latter condition usually causes dysphagia by direct mechanical protrusion and involvement of the posterior aspect of the pharyngoesophagus. It also may compromise the blood supply to the medulla or associated cranial nerves.

Neurodevelopmental Disorders

Numerous neurodevelopmental disorders may affect the normal swallow.
Syringomyelia is a condition of unknown and complex etiology that often occurs early in life. It progresses in the form of an enlarging cystic cavity centrally located in the spinal cord or medulla. When it involves the spinal cord, it is more commonly situated in the region adjacent to the cervical cord. This affects the neural outflow to the upper extremities. Syringomyelia

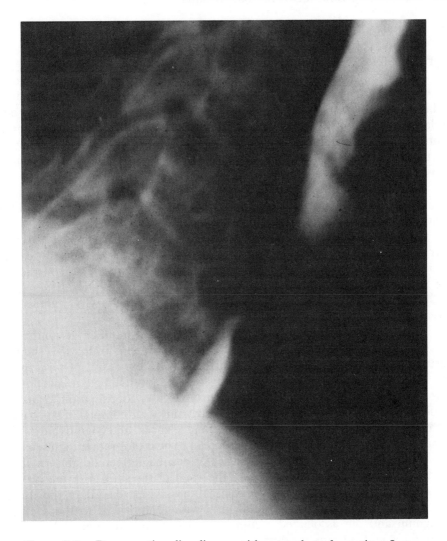

Figure 2.3.   Degenerative disc disease with osteophyte formation. Lateral view of an upper gastrointestinal series using solids impregnated with barium. The column of barium is disrupted by a prominent osteophyte. Reprinted by permission of the publisher and the authors, from Lambert et al., *American Journal of Gastroenterology,* vol. 76, 1981.

(affecting the spinal cord) is less commonly associated with dysphagia than syringobulbia, which affects the medulla or other regions of the brainstem in a similar process, obliterating structures necessary for normal swallowing.

Klippel-Feil syndrome occurs as a result of fusion of cervical vertebrae during embryonic development with a resultant decrease in the length of the cervical spine. This is expressed as shortening of the neck and is accompanied by paraparesis. There may be direct involvement of the medulla as a result of buckling or compression of the brainstem, and there may be associated syringobulbia.

Dandy-Walker syndrome results from prenatal obstruction to the outflow of cerebrospinal fluid through normal apertures in the fourth ventricle. This is accompanied by the development of a cyst in the posterior fossa and dilation of the fourth ventricle and aqueduct, with upward displacement of some brainstem structures and compression of others. Involvement of neural structures subserving swallow depends on the specific abnormalities in a given patient.

Arnold-Chiari syndrome is a congenital abnormality that displaces the hindbrain downward with alteration of relationships of the pons, medulla, and cerebellum. The abnormality may be accompanied by vascular lesions in the tegmentum of the medulla as a result of changes in the vascular arrangement to the herniated portion of the brainstem as the arteries are stretched. In addition to hemorrhages in the medulla, compression or traction of the vagus and other lower cranial nerves may result. Patients may have respiratory distress, apnea, vocal fold paralysis, or inability to swallow (Papasozomenos and Roessmann, 1981).

The term cerebral palsy is used to describe a number of syndromes resulting from defective development of the embryonic brain. The changes usually are not progressive beyond birth, but are the result of teratogenic or other abnormalities occurring during pregnancy. Defects in swallowing often are related to abnormalities in neuromuscular coordination, frank paresis or paralysis of swallowing-related structures, or complex disturbances that may include weakness, incoordination, seizures, and cognitive dysfunction. The predominant abnormalities appear to be motor rather than sensory.

Other neurodevelopmental causes of dysphagia include abnormalities in the growth and resultant angle of the vault of the skull with the cervical spine, called platybasia or basilar invagination. In these disorders, the altered shape and inclination of the skull base with relationship to the foramen magnum and the associated contents results in compression of brainstem structures and subsequent dysphagia.

A malignant form of neurofibromatosis includes many types of recurrent neoplasms of the nervous system, especially neurofibromas (neurinomas), sarcomas, and meningiomas. These may occur in virtually any location, but are of note in relation to swallowing when they involve the brainstem, associated cranial nerves, and/or contiguous bony structures.

PSYCHOGENIC CAUSES OF DEGLUTITION DISORDERS

A number of conditions having primary, predominant, or associated emotional or psychogenic causes may affect swallowing. Since the strict definition of dysphagia requires that "difficulty in swallowing" be encountered during or seconds after the act of swallowing, some of these disorders cannot properly be included under the heading of dysphagia.

Swallowing difficulties that reflect a person's emotional state, coping mechanisms, or responses to life stress may involve other areas of the gastrointestinal tract in a complex fashion. In the case of peptic ulcer or hiatal hernia, a chain of events may result; the dysphagia may be secondary to the effects of stress on the primary disease. In Plummer-Vinson syndrome, several specific abnormalities occur and have been described. In addition to these, achalasia and hiatal hernia may coexist, together with recognizable emotional disturbances that appear to be part of this syndrome. Patients with emotional conversion symptoms who suffer from anxiety may complain of a lump in the throat (globus hystericus), which is extremely uncomfortable but does not appear to interfere with their ability to swallow (Bockus, 1944). Less dramatic responses to stress often are accompanied by prolonged esophageal emptying time (Wolfe and Almy, 1949). It is important that patients with symptoms referable to swallowing that are accompanied by positive features of psychogenic or emotional origin not be denied an appropriate history and physical examination lest a physical or organic cause be overlooked. The relationship between psychogenic dynamics and organic causes was highlighted by Black (1980), who reported treatment by hypnosis of dysphagia following traumatic pseudobulbar palsy.

SUMMARY

It is apparent that the process of moving a bolus from mouth to stomach takes place in an organized fashion only if the necessary neuromuscular and neuroregulatory controls are intact. Perhaps the inherent complexity of the process predisposes its delicately balanced neural control to potential failure from the myriad of disease entities under discussion. Even as this chapter details the neurologic disorders of swallowing, the clinician may feel overwhelmed when confronted with the process of differentially diagnosing swallowing disorders secondary to neurogenic and myogenic causes. It should be apparent that most swallowing dysfunctions are not without cause, and most often are the result of an underlying disease process. For this reason, patients with dysphagic complaints require diagnostic exploration. Discovery of the disease process may be difficult, especially in its beginning stages, as the initial symptoms frequently suggest more than one condition. The difficulty in specifying a particular disease or disorder may not be as important initially as discovering which neuromotor system is involved or at which anatomic level the pathology exists. Although a careful analysis of clinical and laboratory data suggests that this task is immediately feasible, the existence of multiple diagnostic and nosologic entities presenting as apparently identical or similar symptoms constitutes a challenge to clinicians to devise additional reliable tests of the neuromuscular components of swallowing. Completion of such an evaluation should provide the clinician with reasonable assumptions about short- and long-term treatment strategies.

REFERENCES

Bastiaensen LAK, Schulte BPM. Oculopharyngeal dystrophy: diagnostic problems and possibilities. Doc Ophthalmol 1979; 46:391–401.

Black S. Dysphagia of pseudobulbar palsy successfully treated by hypnosis. NZ Med J 1980; 91:212–4.

Bockus HL. Gastroenterology. Philadelphia: W.B. Saunders, 1944.

Bosch EP, Gowans JDC, Munsat T. Oculopharyngeal dystrophy. Muscle Nerve 1979; 2:73–7.

Bosma JF, Brodie DR. Cineradiographic demonstration of pharyngeal area myotonia in myotonic dystrophy patients. Radiology 1969; 92:104–9.

Bramble MG, Cunliffe J, Dellipiani W. Evidence for a change in neurotransmitter affecting esophageal motility in Parkinson's disease. J Neurol Neurosurg Psychiatry 1978; 41:709–12.

Calne DB, Shaw DG, Spiers ASD, Stern GM. Swallowing in Parkinsonism. Br J Radiol 1970; 43:456–7.

Carpenter RJ 3rd, McDonald TJ, Howard FM Jr. The otolaryngologic presentation of amyotrophic lateral sclerosis. Otolaryngology 1978; 86:479–84.

Carter SL. Resolution of postvagal dysphagia. JAMA 1978; 240:2656–57.

Delisa JA, Mikulic MA, Miller RM, Melnick RR. Amyotrophic lateral sclerosis: comprehensive management. Am Fam Physician 1979; 19:137–42.

Duranceau CA, Letendre J, Clermont RJ, Leresque HP, Barbeau A. Oropharyngeal dysphagia in patients with oculopharyngeal muscular dystrophy. Can J Surg 1978; 21:326–9.

Dworkin JP, Hartman DE. Progressive speech deterioration and dysphagia in amyotrophic lateral sclerosis: case report. Arch Phys Med Rehabil 1979; 60:423–5.

Eaton L, Lambert E. Electromyograph and electrical stimulation of nerves in disease of motor unit: observation on myasthenic syndrome associated with malignant tumors. JAMA 1957; 163:1117–21.

Everett NB. Functional neuroanatomy. Philadelphia: Lea and Febiger, 1965.

Fischer RA, Ellison GW, Thayor WR. Esophageal motility in neuromuscular disorders. Ann Intern Med 1965; 63:229–48.

Harvey JC, Sherbourne DH, Siegel CI. Smooth muscle involvement in myotonic dystrophy. Amer J Med 1965; 39:81–90.

Lambert JR, Tepperman P, Jimenez JJ, Newman A. Cervical spine disease and dysphagia. Am J Gastroenterol 1981; 76:35–40.

Latimer PR. Biofeedback and self-regulation in the treatment of diffuse esophageal spasm: a single case study. Biofeedback Self Regul 1981; 6:181–9.

Leclercq TA, DeRobbio AV. Dysphagia secondary to ankylosing vertebral hyperostosis. RI Med J 1978; 61:347–50.

Lieberman AM, Horowitz L, Redmond P, Pachter L, Lieberman I, Leibowitz M. Dysphagia in Parkinson's disease. Am J Gastroenterol 1980; 74:157–60.

Logemann JA, Boshes B, Blonsky ER. Speech and swallowing evaluation in the differential diagnosis of neurologic disease. Neurologica Neurocirugia Psiquiatria 1977; 18:71–8.

Ludman H. Dysphagia in dystrophia myotonica. J Laryngol 1962; 76:234–6.

McGuirt WF, Blalock D. The otolaryngologist's role in the diagnosis and treatment of amyotrophic lateral sclerosis. Laryngoscope 1980; 90:1496–1501.

Metheny JA. Dermatomyositis: a vocal and swallowing disease entity. Laryngoscope 1978; 88:147–61.

Morgan AA, Mourant AJ. Left vocal cord paralysis and dysphagia in mitral valve disease. Br Heart J 1980; 43:470–3.

O'Connor AFF, Ardran GM. Cinefluorography in the diagnosis of pharyngeal palsies. J Laryngol Otol 1976; 90:1015–19.

Pahor AL. Herpes zoster of the larynx—how common? J Laryngol Otol 1979; 93:93–8.

Pallis CA. Parkinsonism: natural history and clinical futures. Br Med J 1971; 3:683–90.

Papasozomenos S, Roessmann U. Respiratory distress and Arnold-Chiari malformation. Neurology 1981; 31:97–100.

Peppercorn MA, Docken WP, Rosenberg S. Esophageal motor dysfunction in systematic lupus erythematosus. JAMA 1979; 242:1895–6.

Pierce JW, Creamer B, MacDermot V. Abnormalities in swallowing associated with dystrophia myotonica. Gut 1965; 6:392–5.

Pope CE. Motor disorders of the esophagus. Postgrad Med 1977; 61:118–25.

Rubenstein AE, Horowitz SH, Bender AN. Cholinergic dysautonomia and Eaton-Lambert syndrome. Neurology 1979; 29:720–3.

Sasaki CT. Paralysis of the larynx and pharynx. Surg Clin North Am 1980; 60:1079–91.

Schultz A, Niemtzow P, Jacobs S, Naso F. Dysphagia associated with cricopharyngeal dysfunction. Arch Phys Med Rehabil 1979; 60:381–6.

Smith AW, Mulder DW, Code CF. Esophageal motility in amyotrophic lateral sclerosis. Mayo Clin Proc 1957; 32:438–41.

Smith RA, Norris FH. Symptomatic care of patients with amyotrophic lateral sclerosis. JAMA 1975; 234:715–7.

Vantrappen G, Janssens J, Hellemans J, Coremans G. Achalasia, diffuse esophageal spasm, and related motility disorders. Gastroenterology 1979; 76:450–7.

Weider DJ, Tingwald FR. Dysphagia as initial and prime symptom of tetanus. Arch Otolaryngol 1970; 91:479–81.

Wolf S, Almy TP. Experimental observations on cardiospasm in man. Gastroenterology 1949; 13:401–21.

CHAPTER 3

Mechanical Disorders of Swallowing
Michael E. Groher

Patients with mechanical swallowing disorders evidence difficulty secondary to the loss of sensory guidance of the structures necessary to complete a normal swallow. The central and most of the peripheral neurologic controls for deglutition are intact. The structures needed to complete the act are not. Even though causes and mechanisms of the neurologic and mechanical groups are different, some of the deglutitory problems are shared. These include sialorrhea (excessive expectoration of fluid resembling saliva), difficulty with mastication, oral and pharyngeal pooling, lengthened swallowing transit times, difficulty channeling food into the esophagus, and aspiration. For the purposes of this and subsequent chapters, aspiration is defined as the residual, unswallowed pharyngeal content that is drawn into the larynx and trachea by inspiration following an attempt at a normal swallow. It is to be differentiated from spillage of oral contents into the pharynx and/or larynx without elicitation of swallow; this is penetration. Most patients with mechanical dysphagia have had oral, pharyngeal, or laryngeal structures removed or reconstructed during surgery for cancer. There are, however, other causes that must be considered in the differential diagnosis. The most common of these are considered here.

ACUTE INFLAMMATIONS

Acute inflammatory processes that produce or exacerbate dysphagia are nonspecific reactions to injury of the oropharyngeal tissue secondary to bacterial or viral agents, chemical irritants, or traumatic insults.

Acute inflammations of the oropharyngeal tissues alone may not create significant, extended dysphagia. They are particularly significant, however, when superimposed on other more obvious swallowing disorders such as pseudobulbar dysphagia or the dysphagia seen in elderly debilitated patients. Early recognition and treatment of acute inflammatory reactions can make the difference between success and failure in attempts at oral feeding. They should be ruled out in patients whose mental state or competence interferes with the ability to communicate oral pain and those who evidence unexplainable dysphagia or sudden refusal to eat. Early identification is important because most such inflammations can be controlled within a short period of time, and oral nutritional intake can resume.

Acute Pharyngitis

Acute pharyngitis may be viral or bacterial in origin. The reddened inflammation that it causes in the oropharyngeal region frequently precedes the common cold, leading patients to complain of swallowing difficulty. It often is accompanied by a mild fever without any other complications. The pain and dysphagia subside within four to six days.

The most common bacterial form of pharyngitis is streptococcal. The diagnosis is confirmed by laboratory analysis. The patient has an acutely inflamed oropharynx with characteristic white or yellow follicles. Most complain of headache and muscle joint pain and have fevers that reach 103 degrees. Streptococcal infections respond well to a full course of antibiotics.

Lingual Tonsillitis

Patients with lingual tonsillitis have symptoms similar to those of other throat infections, except they complain of pain in the medial pharyngeal region. Often they describe a lump in the throat associated with complaints of dysphagia. The mechanism of lingual tonsillitis can be confirmed by indirect mirror examination of the base of the tongue and pharynx.

Herpes Simplex

Viral in origin, a herpetic infection is characterized by round vesicles that break to form shallow ulcers surrounded by a narrow zone of inflammation (DeWeese and Saunders, 1973). Typically, they are found on the lips; however, the pharynx and buccal mucosa may be involved. Palatal and pharyngeal ulcers create significant pain and discomfort on swallowing.

Fungal Inflammation

One of the common fungal inflammations is moniliasis (thrush). Most frequently seen on the tongue, the lesions appear as soft, white, slightly elevated plaques (Keyes, 1980) (Figure 3.1). If left untreated, the lesions cause associated pain and difficulty swallowing. They are more common in debilitated

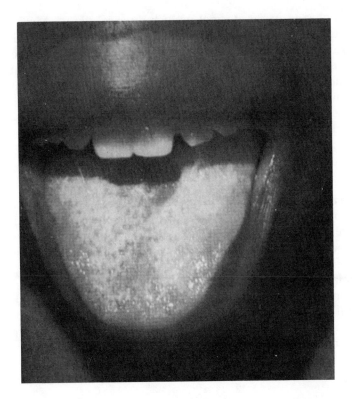

Figure 3.1. Fungal inflammations of the tongue appear as milky-white elevated lesions. Reprinted by permission of the publisher, from Dreizen et al., *Postgrad Med,* 61 1977a.

patients, in those who are undergoing extensive antibiotic therapy, and in patients receiving irradiation treatments. They are differentiated from other white plaques such as leukoplakia because they can be scraped away, leaving a raw bloody surface (Keyes, 1980).

Chemical Agents

Mucosal inflammation may result from exposure to chemicals. The subsequent pain interferes most often with the oropharyngeal stage of swallowing.

Chemical inflammation can result from the prolonged use of phenol (toothache drops). Other drugs that precipitate mucosal burns include aspirin, which causes irritation to the cheek lining, some gargles, and anesthetic throat lozenges when used excessively (Kerr and Ash, 1978). The latter reduce oral sensation and invite traumatic lesions from persons who unknowingly bite their oral mucosa. Mucosal burns can be red or white, but represent a change in the normal pinkish mucosal lining. More severe inflammations have a whitish slough covering an intensely reddened area. The most severe form of a chemical burn, lye ingestion, can cause severe blistering of the entire digestive tract. The clinician should be aware that patients who undergo chemotherapy can develop painful oral ulcerations that interfere with swallowing. Drugs used in these regimens such as doxorubicin (Adriamycin), methotrexate, and cyclophosphamide (Cytoxan) can cause oral mucositis (Carl, 1980).

TRAUMA

Other than major traumatic tissue losses such as those resulting from gunshot wounds, more frequently occurring injuries in the oral cavity are fairly benign and generally do not create significant swallowing complaints except when superimposed on other mechanisms of dysphagia. Examples include trauma from a toothbrush and mucosal irritation from ill-fitting dentures. Patients who complain of a poorly fitted denture can localize their pain. Clinical examination usually will reveal a reddened or whitish change in the mucosa at the point of contact where the patient has the sensation of most discomfort. Prolonged irritation can result in gingival hyperplasia (Figure 3.2) that results in soft, sometimes flexible masses of tissue that appear markedly inflamed.

Biting the sides of the lip, or more commonly, the cheek due to loss of

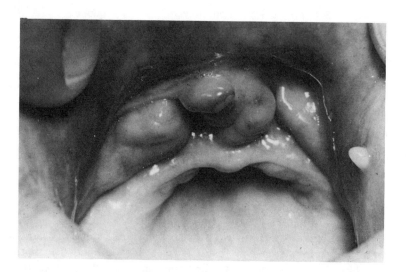

Figure 3.2. Gingival hyperplasia due to an ill-fitting denture. Reprinted by permission of the publisher, from DeWeese and Saunders, *Textbook of otolaryngology*, 6th edition. St. Louis: The C. V. Mosby Co., 1982.

sensation may create some swallowing discomfort. These lesions usually appear as small, irregularly shaped areas covered by a gray necrotic membrane surrounded by inflammation (LaVelle and Proctor, 1978).

MACROGLOSSIA

An abnormally large tongue can interfere with the propulsive action of the bolus. The clinician should be aware of some of the conditions that may contribute to macroglossia that may be considered in the differential diagnosis. They include macroglossia secondary to lymphatic obstruction secondary to surgery or irradiation, hypothyroidism, mongolism, amyloid deposits, and lymphangiomatous or hemangiomatous processes.

MECHANICAL DYSPHAGIA
SECONDARY TO CARCINOMA

The largest group of patients with mechanical swallowing disorders have had oral, pharyngeal, laryngeal, and esophageal structures removed, rearranged, or reconstructed secondary to surgery for carcinoma. Most often, combinations of these structures are involved.

Most clinicians are aware of the general rule for predicting significant dysphagic episodes following surgical excision: if less than 50 percent of an area or organ concerned with deglutition is removed, this will not interfere seriously or permanently with swallowing function (Conley, 1960). A review of the pertinent literature suggests that we must use care when applying this rule.

First, the word "seriously" is nonspecific and can be defined in many different and subjective ways. Second, permanent dysphagia could mean that the patient has persistent dysphagia and cannot tolerate oral feedings, or it could mean that there will be difficulty initiating or completing a normal swallow, but oral feedings will be tolerated with limited success if supplemented by alternative methods. Differences in the permanence of the disorders suggest different treatment approaches and final outcomes. In short, the 50 percent rule is only a guide, and individual differences should not be overlooked. In fact, individual differences among patients who have had cancerous lesions and subsequent resections may not be related to the amount of the structure removed, but to factors such as preoperative and postoperative health, psychologic reaction to the disability, and ability to learn adaptive swallowing techniques.

The 50 percent rule also applies if the structure in question is rearranged, or if adjacent structures are rearranged (Summers, 1974; Weaver and Fleming, 1978). Procedures on adjacent structures appear to carry a more negative prognosis for deglutitory recovery than does loss of mobility of those structures (Doberneck and Antoine, 1974).

Sessions and co-workers (1979) implied that the 50 percent rule not be applied randomly to any swallowing structure. They pointed out that the original size of the lesion was not as important a prognosticator of dysphagia as was the area excised, and that resultant dysphagia could be predicted if surgical excision involved either the arytenoid cartilages or the base of the tongue. Logemann and Bytell (1979) analyzed swallowing transit times and motility in three separate groups of patients with head and neck resections. They concluded, "We cannot assume that the patient facing less ablative surgery will have only minimal functional problems in swallowing." Although this conclusion appears to stand alone, the differences in data interpretation once again come from how we define a minimal as opposed to a significant swallowing disorder. In fact, the overall success at oral feeding during and after the study period was not reported in the Logemann and Bytell (1979) data. Therefore, it is difficult to interpret the ultimate significance of dysphagia in those patients who have abnormal videofluoroscopic findings with little ablative surgery.

An additional complication to the loss of structural function is the total or partial loss of sensation, or interruption of the neurologic afferent controls in the oropharynx that surgical procedures can precipitate. The use of tissue flaps to close surgical defects interferes with the normal sensation that provides adequate sensory guidance of the bolus needed to effect a normal swallow.

In addition to receiving surgical treatment for lesions, patients also may be candidates for irradiation in an effort to control the malignancy. There is agreement among clinicians that preoperative or postoperative irradiation predisposes the patient to dysphagic complications more than if this treatment were not undertaken (Summers, 1974; Weaver and Fleming, 1978; Sessions, Zill, and Schwartz, 1979).

EXPECTED IMPAIRMENT FROM SURGICAL RESECTIONS

Following this introduction to mechanical deglutition disorders secondary to carcinoma, the impairment that can be expected from the most common types of resections is reviewed.

Oral Lesions

Cancers in the oral cavity may involve the tongue, floor of the mouth and submental structures, tonsils, soft palate (velum), mandible, and maxilla.

Many times, more than one of these structures is involved. It is not unusual to have parts of the tongue, mandible, and floor of the mouth resected.

In general, patients with resected oral structures have difficulty with mastication, formation and retention of a bolus, and anteroposterior transport. Major resections of parts of the mandible and submental region can significantly alter the relationships among oral, pharyngeal, and laryngeal structures, resulting in disburbance of the sequential movements involved in swallowing. For instance, loss of the occlusal jaw relationships after mandibulectomy can interfere with mastication in such a way as to lengthen the oral phase of feeding. This can result not only in delayed and therefore poorly timed propulsion, but in premature attempts at swallowing because the delay is not well tolerated by most patients.

Patients with resections that involve the tongue (glossectomy) experience difficulty with bolus transport to the oropharynx. The question of how much this delay in schedule permanently interferes with the oral route of feeding remains somewhat controversial; most evidence supports the fact that even patients who lose all of their tongue can swallow.

After reviewing over 700 patients with resected tongue lesions (some had had preoperative irradiation), Frazell and Lucas (1962) reported that 40 of the 168 patients experienced transitory dysphagic complications, and only 13 of the 168 required permanent tube feedings. Other investigators have reported similar success, although most describe periods of transitory postoperative dysphagia that is dependent partially on the amount of tongue that is resected. Frazell and Lucas (1962) implied that the prognosis for recovery of swallow was better for those who did not have structures other than the tongue resected, such as part of the mandible or the submental region. They concluded that postoperative complications were correlated more positively with preoperative factors such as age and general health, size and position of the primary tumor, invasion of neighboring structures, and status of the regional lymph nodes.

Conley (1960) and Summers (1974) agreed that patients who lose up to one-third of the tongue have only transitory swallowing disorders. These resolve in two to four weeks without specific remediation of dysphagia.

Patients who undergo glossectomy that includes the base of the tongue are susceptible to persistent dysphagia, although the majority can successfully eat orally. Donaldson, Skelly, and Paletta (1968) reported that 8 of 14 patients with total glossectomy had no dysphagia, while the remaining 6 had to rely on tube feedings. One of the six eventually had to undergo elective total laryngectomy to control the dysphagia. Myers (1972) reported a higher swallowing success rate in a series of 14 patients following glossectomy, all but one of whom were able to take nutrition orally. Summers (1974) noted that the majority of patients with glossectomy do well following surgery because they are able to protect their airway with an intact laryngeal sphincter.

Logemann and Bytell (1979) provided a more detailed analysis of the deglutition problems glossectomy patients might encounter one week after attempts at oral feeding. They studied by videofluoroscopy ten patients who had excision of lesions of the floor of the mouth and tongue (10 to 70 percent of those structures) with accompanying dissections of the anterior mandible and neck. All had difficulty forming and maintaining a bolus. Oral transit times were delayed, except in the two patients who had longitudinally divided tongue flaps. Eight of the patients were unable to chew because they could not orient material to the molar table. All experienced difficulty with anterior drooling. The swallowing stimuli (thin barium, cookie coated with barium paste, cookie with thin barium) often collected in the anterior and lateral sulci. Oral content of thick consistency was accumulated on the oral palate. Anteroposterior propulsion was disturbed and the bolus frequently spilled into the oropharynx before the patient was ready to initiate a swallow. This was true for all food consistencies used, except for the thin paste that required less oral effort and was associated with better transport times. Once the bolus was moved posteriorly, all patients could initiate a swallow.

Kothary and DeSouza (1973) used cineradiography in their analysis of 25 patients undergoing glossectomy. They found that these patients compensated well for poor lingual propulsion by increasing the use of the buccal musculature, inclining the floor of the mouth, and more prominent forward movement of the pharyngeal musculature.

Even though these problems exist in the early postoperative stages, reports in the literature suggest that patients with tongue resections uncomplicated by surgical involvement of related structures are able to take nutrition orally after no longer than a one-month period of adjustment to their disability. Unfortunately, a significant number of patients must undergo resection of structures of more than the tongue to achieve adequate control of the cancer.

Summers (1974) found that patients with these composite resections required weeks or months to relearn swallowing, and that there usually is a much more pronounced degree of frustration with eating than for those who have had only glossectomy. Conley (1960) supported this observation by noting that patients who had a hemiglossectomy with floor of the mouth, adjacent mandible, and ipsilateral neck dissection did recover the ability to swallow, but with some aspiration, coughing, and anxiety associated with swallowing attempts.

Patients who must undergo glossectomy and submental resections not only may lose tongue propulsion and lip sensation, but the protective tilting action of the larynx provided by the hypomandibular constrictors is sacrificed. This can result in significant aspiration. Conley (1960) reported that patients who had undergone total glossectomy with bilateral dissections of cervical lymph nodes swallowed poorly, but if both superior laryngeal nerves, the hyoid, and epiglottis were intact, they could swallow a liquid diet without aspiration.

Patients with resections of the tongue, neck, floor of the mouth, and mandible (Figure 3.3) have different degrees of dysphagia impairment: of the masticatory process, bolus control, and anteroposterior propulsion. Reconstruction of the structures in the mandibular region can create scar tissue contractures and temporomandibular joint pain interfering with normal mastication (Figure 3.4). Not only is it difficult to place food due to limited excursion, but subsequent swallows may be poorly timed because of abnormal occlusal relationships. These poor mandibular/maxillary contacts make

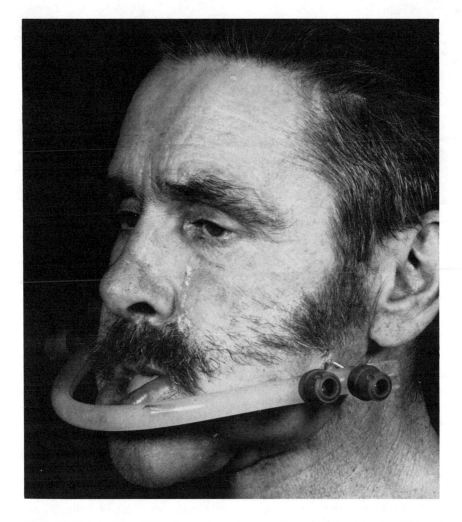

Figure 3.3. Patient following surgery for carcinoma of the anterior floor of the mouth and mandible with a right radical and left suprahyoid resection including the tongue. A right trapezius myocutaneous flap was used to reconstruct the oral cavity and a biphase appliance was used to temporarily fixate the mandible.

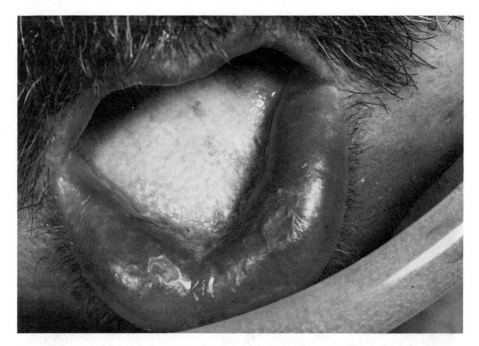

Figure 3.4.   Floor of the mouth of the patient in Figure 3.3. Absence of a mobile tongue and a lower immobile lip made anterior/posterior propulsion difficult.

biting and chewing more of an effort and tend to interfere with bolus formation.

Partial Laryngectomy

Partial laryngectomy is a general category of surgical resection of the pharyngeal and laryngeal region that seeks to control a malignancy while preserving vocal function and deglutition. These procedures are principally hemilaryngectomy and supraglottic laryngectomy.

Hemilaryngectomy

Definitions vary on what constitutes a hemilaryngectomy. Leonard, Holt, and Maran (1972) defined it as unilateral excision of the vocal fold plus extension to the anterior commissure or the vocal processes, or both. Weaver and Fleming's (1978) definition includes unilateral resection of the vocal fold, vestibular fold, ventricle, and superior laryngeal nerve with preservation of the epiglottis. The present discussion uses the latter definition. The typical resection that comprises a hemilaryngectomy is illustrated in Figure 3.5.

Weaver and Fleming (1978) studied a group of 11 patients undergoing

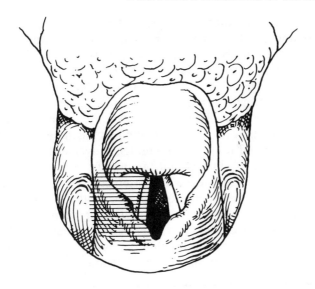

Figure 3.5. Hemilaryngectomy defines an anatomic defect which typically includes the true and
false cords and aryepiglottic fold unilaterally. The
ipsilateral superior laryngeal nerve is removed
while the epiglottis is spared. Reprinted by permission of the publisher, from Weaver and Fleming, *Amer J Surg,* 1978.

hemilaryngectomy at periods of six weeks and six months postresection. The
results showed that 7 of 11 had no swallowing difficulty with solids or liquids
at either evaluation. Two patients had initial problems that resolved at six
months, one failed to swallow adequately after six months, and one had
recurrence of disease. The only patient who did not recover swallow had
preoperative irradiation, neck dissection, and a postoperative fistula.

Leonard et al. (1972) found similarly encouraging results. Of the 75
patients with excised unilateral lesions that had not extended significantly,
aspiration was not a problem except in those who already were debilitated
and also had poor pulmonary function. None of the 75 had an immobile
vocal fold prior to surgery. The authors implied that this may have contributed significantly to their good results.

The results reported by Schoenrock and associates (1972) were less
encouraging. After unilaterally severing and elevating the infrahyoid muscles
to form a perichondrial muscle pedicle flap, the thyroid ala, arytenoid, and
vestibular and vocal folds were removed. In addition, the ipsilateral superior
laryngeal nerve was sectioned and the pyriform sinus obliterated. Seven of
the 11 patients who were studied two months postoperatively aspirated thin
barium; one aspirated thick barium. Of the seven patients, only three subjectively complained of aspiration. Schoenrock's group (1972) attributed

their findings to the fact that the larynx did not rise evenly on the excised side. This created a tilting of the larynx that directed the barium to the resected side, eventually spilling into the trachea. Cineradiography showed seven patients' larynges failed to meet the base of the tongue on the excised side during the swallow, thus offering limited protection against penetration into the trachea. In addition, normal sequential pharyngeal constriction was absent on the involved side, further contributing to aspiration. These authors noted that all seven patients had incompetent glottal chinks. Four of the seven could not achieve enough movement to get closure and three had good movement, but the functioning true vocal fold met the excised mucosal surface at a different level. It is interesting to note that even though aspiration in some of these patients was not subjectively apparent, it was demonstrated by chest radiography. This finding seemed to suggest that patients may be asymptomatic for a long period of time and then develop pulmonary complications, including minimal basilar pneumonia, pulmonary fibrosis, multiple lobe aspiration, aspiration pneumonia, and lung abscess.

Supraglottic Laryngectomy

Supraglottic laryngectomy has several definitions. Weaver and Fleming (1978) defined it as a resection that "typically includes both false cords, both aryepiglottic folds, and one or both superior laryngeal nerves." Summers (1974) defined the resection as a "block resection of the vallecula, epiglottis, hyoid bone, aryepiglottic folds, ventricular bands, upper third of the thyroid cartilage, and thyrohyoid membrane." Flores and co-workers (1982) agreed with Summers and included the pre-epiglottic space. They pointed out that some supraglottic resections extend to include the resection of one arytenoid, the pyriform sinus (partial laryngopharyngectomy), and/or the base of the tongue. The careful reader will note the potential differences in data interpretation relative to supraglottic resections as different criteria for patient selection may bias the results. For the purposes of this discussion, a supraglottic laryngectomy includes resection of both vestibular and aryepiglottic folds and one or both superior laryngeal nerves (Weaver and Fleming, 1978) (Figure 3.6).

Most investigators agree that supraglottic resections are not without dysphagic complications, especially in the immediate (two- to four-week) postoperative period. The eventual severity and duration beyond this period appears to be highly variable, however, partly due to the fact that not all supraglottic resections remove identical structures, some patients develop postsurgical complications, and some receive either preoperative or postoperative irradiation. While a small majority eventually do swallow with minimal aspiration, resections that compromise the arytenoids and extend into the pyriform sinus and tongue base create significant and sometimes persisting dysphagia (Conley, 1960; Staple and Ogura, 1966; Litton and Leonard, 1969; Summers, 1974; Weaver and Fleming, 1978; Flores et al.,

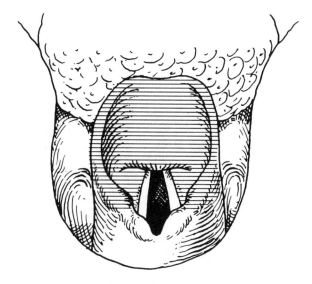

Figure 3.6. Bilateral supraglottic laryngectomy describes removal of the entire supraglottis. Hopefully, one superior laryngeal nerve can be preserved. Reprinted by permission of the publisher, from Weaver and Fleming, *Amer J Surg*, 1978.

1982). Loss of the tongue base apparently impairs glottic protection as the larynx is elevated. Loss of arytenoid masses also results in impairment of the glottis at the laryngeal level.

Sacrificing one superior laryngeal nerve (SLN) during supraglottic resection does not significantly interfere with swallowing, although bilateral excision carries a negative prognosis for pharyngeal deglutition (Shedd, 1976; Weaver and Fleming, 1978). Bocca, Pignataro, and Mosciaro (1968) and Flores et al. (1982) did not find that bilateral excision of the superior laryngeal nerve influenced the severity or duration of dysphagia. In fact, the latter group reported that immediate success at deglutition (as a proportional percentage) was higher with bilateral SLN resections, although this was not statistically significant. They pointed out that this variable "probably should not be considered separately since preservation of one SLN is related to the preservation of the hyoid bone." Their patients with hyoid resections had a better prognosis for swallowing.

Weaver and Fleming (1978) measured swallowing competence of 23 patients following unilateral and bilateral supraglottic resections at six weeks and six months after surgery. All 23 had difficulty with both liquids and solids. After six months, 16 still had dysphagia that ranged from mild to persistent. The most severely affected patients also had had resections of the tongue base. Not one of the four who underwent bilateral supraglottic resections regained their normal swallow, although three were able to maintain their weight with acceptable levels of aspiration (e.g., no pulmonary complications). The one patient who had persistent aspiration had both superior laryngeal nerves severed and also had postoperative irradiation.

Staple and Ogura (1966) followed 36 patients with supraglottic laryngectomy who had excision of the epiglottis, both aryepiglottic folds and the pre-epiglottic space, vestibular folds, upper one-third of the thyroid cartilage on the affected side, and a smaller segment on the unaffected side. One-half of the 36 had initial periods of barium aspiration but regained their swallowing function so that oral nutrition could be maintained. Five patients evidenced persistent dysphagia but did well after one to two years. This led the authors to remark on the potential adaptability of the surgically interrupted swallowing mechanism. Because half of this group did experience some mild aspiration, a follow-up study (Staple, Ragsdale, and Ogura, 1967) was done to assess the long-term effects on the lungs of mild aspiration. Chest films were taken at four months and an average of two and one-half years after surgery. At four months, 14 of the 27 patients reviewed had pneumonia. At two years, 13 of the 39 studied had pneumonia. The authors concluded that although patients who aspirated during these measurements had a poor prognosis for recovery of deglutition, the outcome was, in most cases, not fatal.

Flores and co-workers (1982) studied those particular factors that might correlate with success in oral deglutition in 46 patients following supraglottic laryngeal surgery. Most of the 46 received high-dose preoperative irradiation. All underwent a typical (Weaver and Fleming, 1978) procedure. Some had additional resections, including the arytenoid, pyriform sinus, and tongue base. Twenty-eight patients were able to rely solely on oral intake within five days after removal of the nasogastric tube. Nine experienced delayed recovery, but could rely solely on oral intake after four weeks to five months. Nine patients failed to swallow. The authors reported that age did not seem to be an important factor in predicting recovery, nor did preservation of the superior larynx or hyoid. Of the 15 patients in whom one arytenoid was sacrificed, a higher proportion (47 percent) failed to swallow than when both were preserved. Partial laryngopharyngectomy carried a negative prognosis for swallowing, although the most successful outcome in this group was in the only patient with preserved arytenoid function.

Logemann and Bytell (1979) studied eight patients with supraglottic laryngectomy with resections ranging from 10 to 50 percent of the tongue base. Fifty percent of the patients aspirated, with test materials falling diffusely into the pharynx in 75 to 92 percent. Laryngeal constriction was limited in one-half of the patients. This group also had some slowing of oral and pharyngeal transit times when compared with healthy persons.

Of 24 patients undergoing traditional and more extensive supraglottic resections, 16 aspirated thick barium paste, although in none was swallow incapacitated (Litton and Leonard, 1969). Cineradiography revealed that 13 of the 16 had barium trapped over the laryngeal inlet and could not clear it on repeated attempts. All 16 who aspirated had pharyngeal involvement in addition to the supraglottic resection. Six also underwent tongue resections. The eight who did not aspirate all evidenced elevation of the laryngeal remnant and none had a resection that involved the pharyngeal wall.

Bocca's group (1968) reported on 223 cases of classic supraglottic resection. No patient received irradiation and only six experienced dysphagia incident to poor arytenoid movement. In the majority of cases, dysphagia subsided within three weeks. Of 192 patients who received irradiation only for treatment of supraglottic lesions, this therapy did not produce significant dysphagia in any (Fayos, 1975).

There are numerous conclusions that become apparent when assessing the potential effects on deglutition following supraglottic laryngectomy. First, patients who undergo the classic resection without bilateral denervation of the superior laryngeal nerve experience mild and transitory dysphagia (Staple and Ogura, 1966; Bocca et al., 1968; Weaver and Fleming, 1978). If the resection extends into the pyriform sinus, pharynx, or the tongue base, approximately one-half of patients have moderate to severe dysphagia, but may be able to tolerate limited oral feedings (Staple and Ogura, 1966; Litton and Leonard, 1969; Logemann and Bytell, 1979).

Second, patients who do best after supraglottic resections have the following characteristics: a mobile tongue base (Staple and Ogura, 1966; Shedd, 1976; Weaver and Fleming, 1978; Sessions et al., 1979), a larynx that rises far enough to meet the tongue base (Bocca et al., 1968; Litton and Leonard, 1969), a resected hyoid bone (Flores et al., 1982), and a glottis that allows for bilateral approximation of the vocal fold (Staple and Ogura, 1966; Summers, 1974; Sessions et al., 1979; Flores et al., 1982). Support for myotomy (surgical relaxation of the cricopharyngeus muscle) at the time of surgery as a procedure to prevent aspiration is provided by Staple and Ogura (1976), rejected by Weaver and Fleming (1978), and is thought to be useful when the hyoid or arytenoid cartilage must be sacrificed (Bocca et al., 1967). Myotomy produces more immediate successful swallowing, but is not effective postoperatively in assisting patients who do not swallow well following supraglottic resection (Flores et al., 1982). Summers (1974) felt the myotomy should be considered in patients expected to have significant postoperative sialorrhea.

Laryngectomy

Even though the alimentary and respiratory tracts are separated surgically, patients undergoing total laryngectomy still are at risk of dysphagia complications, especially in the acute stages of recovery. As might be expected, most of these focus on the physiologic changes the surgery might produce on the cricopharyngeus muscle. Early reports (Schobinger, 1958) concluded that postoperative dysphagia was the result of the cricopharyngeus muscle in spasm. More recent investigations have shown that the cricopharyngeus fails to perform, but not necessarily in a spasmodic fashion.

Using manometrics, Hanks and colleagues (1981) concluded that following laryngectomy the cricopharyngeus was not spastic, but weaker. Summers (1974) pointed out that in the absence of stricture at this level, the cricopharyngeus performs in an incoordinated manner because of detached inferior constrictor muscles. Summers and Kirchner and colleagues (1963) are in agreement that the changes in cricopharyngeal function create a pharyngeal pseudodiverticulum that, in turn, may become the source of regurgitation. Such pseudodiverticula are found at the base of the tongue and in the posterior pharyngeal wall.

Following laryngectomy, the percentage of patients with postsurgical chronic dysphagia is poorly documented. In one study, five of ten patients developed dysphagia (Duranceau et al., 1976). Based on manometrics, all ten were found to have marked derangements in the upper esophageal sphincter.

Kirchner and Scatliff (1962) used cineradiography to examine 43 laryngectomized patients for dysphagia at differing periods of time following surgery. Of the 26 examined immediately postoperatively, they found 12 had dysphagia. Eight of the 12 had fistulas and 4 did not. Even though the majority of the 43 eventually could take their nutrition orally, some had anterior pouch formation with regurgitation, constant accumulation of food and mucus, and complaints of a foreign body sensation.

In a follow-up study, Kirchner and co-workers (1963) examined 35 patients with laryngectomy. They found that dysphagia was caused by a pharyngeal pseudodiverticulum resulting from separation of the pharyngeal suture line at its junction with the tongue base or by uncoordinated contraction of the detached pharyngeal muscles in the absence of stricture.

There is some evidence to suggest that a higher percentage of the laryngectomized patients who also receive irradiation experience dysphagia. Three of the five patients examined by Duranceau and colleagues (1976) had postoperative dysphagia. Hanks et al. (1981) studied ten patients who were dysphagic following laryngectomy, seven of whom had received irradiation. This led the authors to conclude that although this number was small, irradiation may adversely influence upper esophageal motility.

My own experience and that of Weaver and Fleming (1978) suggest that the large majority of those undergoing laryngectomy who have no medical complications swallow normally after ten days and that irradiation retards this recovery in a small number of patients. Forty-seven of 59 laryngectomized patients reported postoperative dysphagia, but all were taking their nutrition orally after discharge from the hospital (Volin, 1980). Only one had persistent dysphagia. There was no significant correlation between preoperative and/or postoperative irradiation and dysphagia.

Jung and Adams (1980) did a retrospective review of 226 laryngectomized patients. Of this group 36 (16 percent) experienced dysphagia; 16 had benign pharyngeal stricture, 14 with stricture due to recurrence; 4 had malignant esophageal cancer; and 2 had benign lower esophageal stricture. The majority had preoperative irradiation. Most of those who experienced dysphagia had laryngopharyngectomy. The authors suggested that the complaint of persistent dysphagia may be a sign of early recurrence, especially if the postpharyngeal space is wider than normal, or if patients have benign strictures.

Irradiation and Deglutition

It is not infrequent for patients who undergo conservative surgical resections for carcinoma also to receive either preoperative or postoperative irradiation, which produces many potential side effects that may further compromise swallowing. They include oral and pharyngeal inflammation with subsequent pain in the soft tissues and bone, a drying effect on the mucosal tissues, diminished volume and thicker consistency of saliva, changes in taste sensation, and loss of appetite. Not all patients experience these symptoms, but when they do, the severity and duration of effects on deglutition are highly variable (Dreizen et al., 1977a).

Loss of Saliva Flow

If irradiation is directed toward the salivary glands in sufficient amounts, patients experience a marked reduction of salivary flow. These changes tend to be permanent and irreversible (Frank et al., 1953; Dreizen et al., 1977b). Of 42 patients with oral cancers who received 260 rads per day, five days a week, salivary flow rates after mastication dropped to 57 percent after the first week, 76 percent after six weeks, and to 95 percent three years after irradiation (Dreizen et al., 1977b).

Hansen, Meyer, and Werner (1970) studied the subjective complaints of 80 patients receiving irradiation for oral lesions. Seventy-eight percent experienced xerostomia during the second week of treatment. This complaint ranked first in a list of six. After six weeks the same individuals were troubled by xerostomia, and after three months it continued to be their major complaint.

When the salivary glands can no longer produce a normal mixture of serous and mucous saliva, deglutition is affected in two ways besides xerostomia: increased dental caries due to loss of the natural defense against decay, and accumulation of stringy mucus that has lost its lubricating abilities (Carl, 1980).

Dental caries create pain during mastication if left untreated (Dreizen et al., 1977b; Weaver and Fleming, 1978). Decay can begin on any tooth and progresses rapidly toward destruction of the dental crown (Dreizen et al., 1977a) (Figure 3.7). Accumulation of thick mucus can in itself mechan-

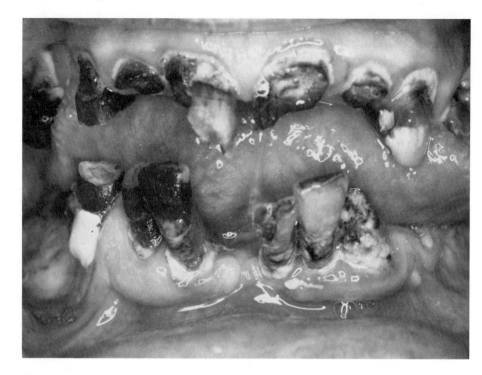

Figure 3.7.   Xerostomia-related dental decay two years after radiotherapy in a patient with cancer of the tongue.

ically interfere with swallowing (Figure 3.8). Hansen and colleagues (1970) found that an accumulation of stringy mucus was the second most common complaint (59 percent) after two and six weeks of irradiation. Patients reported that they were most uncomfortable when the dryness and thick mucus were at their highest point on the twelfth day of radiotherapy. These thick secretions also interfere with denture retention, tissue tolerance to the denture, and taste (Summers, 1974).

Mucositis

Irradiation can produce significant inflammatory changes in the mucous lining, resulting in tenderness and burning not unlike a severe sore throat. A more marked form of these complaints may surface as mucositis (Figure 3.9). When the pain spreads to the pharyngeal mucosa, swallowing can be difficult. This discomfort is antagonized by coarse and highly seasoned foods. Hansen's group (1970) found that 33 percent of their patients complained that inflamed mucosa impeded swallowing. Three months following irradiation, patients no longer had this complaint. Dreizen et al. (1977a) reported

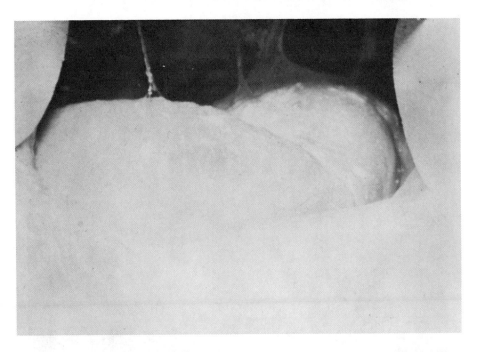

Figure 3.8. Patient with thick mucous secretions secondary to radiotherapy following resection of cancer of the tongue.

that mucositis gradually improved spontaneously three weeks following termination of radiotherapy. Oral mucositis may also result from the use of chemotherapeutic agents such as adriamycin, methotrexate, and cyclophosphamide (Carl, 1980).

Osteoradionecrosis

Osteoradionecrosis can result from oral mucosal destruction at the primary site of irradiation. Developing fibrosis and reduction of blood supply result in the formation of necrotic ulcers that if left untreated can invade bony structures through infectious processes. Ulcers can develop two to three months after radiotherapy or any time thereafter (Dreizen et al., 1977a). The resultant pain can impair oral feeding actions and swallowing to the point at which patients are not able to take nutrition orally. Patients are most vulnerable to osteoradionecrosis of the jaws during the two years following irradiation (Dreizen et al., 1977a). A clinical example is presented in Figure 3.10.

Trismus

Patients who have difficulty with mastication in the form of tonic spasms following or during irradiation may be suffering from trismus. If these mus-

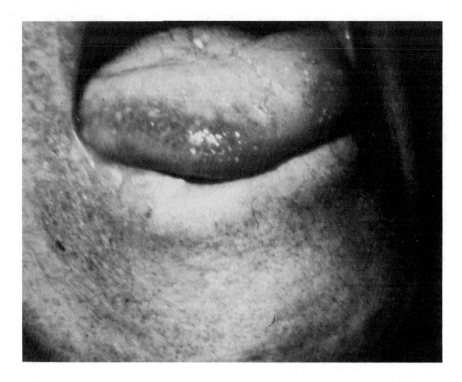

Figure 3.9.   Early radiation mucositis of the tongue in a patient treated for cancer of the floor of the mouth. Reprinted by permission of the publisher, from Dreizen et al., *Postgrad Med* 61, 1977a.

cles are included in the treatment field, jaw excursions may be painful and limited. This is thought to be secondary to masticatory muscle fibrosis.

Loss of Taste and Appetite

Hansen and associates (1970) reported that 53 percent of their patients experienced loss of appetite during and shortly after irradiation. Twenty-two percent said that this was due to a loss of taste, while the remaining 78 percent felt it was related to feelings of nausea and a general dissatisfaction with their diet. Patients generally recover taste acuity 20 to 60 days following radiotherapy, however, and it fully returns after 120 days (Dreizen et al., 1977a). Others have reported specific losses of sweet, salt, and bitter tastes (Conger, 1973, DeWys and Walters, 1975). Aversions to meat and vegetable proteins have also been noted (Fleming, Weaver, and Brown, 1977). Such aversions can lead to loss of appetite, disinterest in food, and eventually, to poor nutrition. Severe loss of proteins, calories, vitamins, and minerals can lead to a nutritional deficiency type of stomatitis.

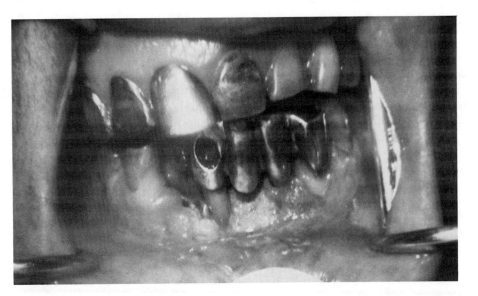

Figure 3.10. Osteoradionecrosis of the mandibular alveolar bone in a patient treated for cancer of the tongue. Reprinted by permission of the publisher, from Dreizen et al., *Postgrad Med* 61, 1977a.

CERVICAL SPINE DISEASE

Osteophytic changes in the cervical spine that put undue mechanical pressure on the esophagus and related structures must be considered in the differential diagnosis of mechanical dysphagia.

Although pressure on the esophagus from the cervical spine is rare (Umerah, Mukherjee, and Ibekur, 1981), other investigators feel that it may just be overlooked as a potential cause and therefore is not as rare as once believed (Lambert et al., 1981). Pressure from cervical osteophytes can be visualized radiographically. Typically, it is found in elderly patients with cervical spondylosis (Umerah et al., 1981) and usually is seen at the level of C4 to C7 (Lambert et al., 1981). Patients complain of pain at the cricopharyngeal level probably due to the pressure of food on the osteophytes (Umerah et al., 1981). All patients complain that solids are harder to swallow than liquids (Lambert et al., 1981). A review of the history of spinal diseases and dysphagia is provided by Gamache and Voorhies (1980).

TRACHEOSTOMA TUBES

Tracheostoma tubes create a mechanical interference to swallowing by restricting normal laryngeal elevation. Loss of elevation compromises glottal protection and invites aspiration. Butcher (1982) reported that tracheostoma tubes increase the chances of aspiration by fixing the larynx anteriorly and preventing its axial rotation. Arms, Dines, and Tinstman (1974) demonstrated that one is at a greater risk for aspiration if a tracheostoma tube is in place.

Bonanno (1971) attempted to investigate the theory that tracheostoma tubes could contribute to dysphagia. He studied 43 patients who underwent elective or semi-elective tracheostomy for general surgery. All were considered to be poor pulmonary risks for general anesthesia. None had head or neck cancer. Previous medical health was not reported. Three of the 43 had postoperative dysphagia because, Bonanno felt, the tracheostoma tube appeared to be anchoring the trachea to the pretracheal strap muscles and the skin of the neck, thus limiting anterior elevation and rotation. Lack of this movement interfered with relaxation of the cricopharyngeus.

It has been my experience that the incidence of dysphagia is greater in patients who have tracheostomy combined with surgical resection of the head and neck. In these cases, patients already have compromised deglutition, and the tracheostoma tube serves as an additional barrier to normal laryngeal elevation.

Patients who have cuffed tracheostoma tubes that are overinflated run the risk of esophageal obstruction from the pressure on the tracheoesophageal wall. The obstruction keeps nutrition from entering the esophagus easily, creating spillover and possible aspiration.

An additional complication is that the presence of the tube prevents expiratory air from being shunted superiorly, resulting in a decrease of expired air needed to clear the larynx after swallowing (Weaver and Fleming, 1982). This reduction of the ability to clear the airway because of mechanical interference may impede rehabilitation (see Chapter 7).

SUMMARY

Mechanical swallowing dysfunction usually is the result of the oral and/or pharyngeal structures being surgically removed or altered. This impairs the displacement of food in the mouth and the bolus in the pharynx. Even though some patients have adequate sensory and motor components for oral and pharyngeal feeding postoperatively, most have significant dysphagia. Additionally, the majority have adequate cortical skills needed for the rehabilitation of feeding.

The dysphagia liability is increased by radiotherapy and/or chemotherapy. A careful evaluation of the pathology as discussed should assist the clinician in working out the diagnostic dilemmas that these patients often present. Treatment suggestions are provided in detail in Chapter 7.

REFERENCES

Arms RA, Dines DE, Tinstman TC. Aspiration pneumonia. Chest 1974;65:136–139.

Bocca E, Pignataro O, Mosciaro O. Supraglottic surgery of the larynx. Ann Otol Rhinol Laryngol 1968;77:1005–26.

Bonanno PC. Swallowing dysfunction after tracheostomy. Ann Surg 1971;174:29–33.

Butcher BR. Treatment of chronic aspiration as a complication of cerebrovascular accident. Laryngoscope 1982;92:681–85.

Carl W. Dental management of head and neck cancer patients. J Surg Oncol 1980;15:265–81.

Conger AD. Loss and recovery of taste acuity in patients irradiated to the oral cavity. Radiat Res 1973;53:338–47.

Conley JJ. Swallowing dysfunctions associated with radical surgery of the head and neck. Arch Surg 1960;80:602–12.

DeWeese DD, Saunders WH. Textbook of otolaryngology. St. Louis: C V Mosby, 1973.

DeWys WD, Walters K. Abnormalities of taste sensation in cancer patients. Cancer 1975;36:1888–96.

Doberneck R, Antoine A. Deglutition after resection of oral, laryngeal and pharyngeal cancers. Surgery 1974;75:87–90.

Donaldson RC, Skelly M, Paletta FX. Total glossectomy for cancer. Am J Surg 1968;116:585–90.

Dreizen S, Daly TE, Drane JB, Brown LR. Oral complications of cancer radiotherapy. Postgrad Med 1977a;61:85–92.

Dreizen S, Brown LR, Daly TE, Drane JB. Prevention of xerostomia-related dental caries in irradiated cancer patients. J Dent Res 1977b;56:99–104.

Duranceau A, Jamieson G, Hurwitz A, Jones L, Scott R, Postlethwait RW. Alteration in esophageal motility after laryngectomy. Am J Surg 1976;131:30–35.

Fayos JV. Carcinoma of the endolarynx: results of irradiation. Cancer 1975;35:1525–32.

Fleming SM, Weaver AW. Clinical management of dysphagia in head and neck cancer patients. Dysarthria, Dysphonia, Dysphagia 1982;1:80–84.

Flores TC, Wood BG, Koegel L Jr, Levine HC, Tucker HM. Factors in successful deglutition following supraglottic laryngeal surgery. Ann Otol Rhinol Laryngol 1982;91:579–83.

Frazell EL, Lucas JC. Cancer of the tongue: report of the management of 1,554 patients. Cancer 1962;15:1085–99.

Gamache FW, Voorhies RM. Hypertrophic cervical osteophytes causing dysphagia. J Neurosurg 1980;53:338–44.

Hanks JB, Fisher SR, Myers WC, Christian KC, Postlethwait RW, Jones RS. Effect of total laryngectomy on esophageal motility. Ann Otol Rhinol Laryngol 1981;90:331–34.

Hansen D, Meyer E, Werner H. Function disorders in the oral cavity as a side effect of radiotherapy. Z Laryngol Rhinol Otol 1970;49:534–41.

Jung TT, Adams GL. Dysphagia in laryngectomized patients. Otolaryngol Head Neck Surg 1980;88:25–33.

Kerr DA, Ash MM. Oral pathology. Philadelphia: Lea & Febiger, 1978.

Keyes KS. Oral mucosal diseases. In: Paparella MM, Shumrick DA, eds. Otolaryngology: head and neck. Philadelphia: W B Saunders, 1980;2136–47.

Kirchner JA, Scatliff JH. Disabilities resulting from healed salivary fistula. Arch Otolaryngol 1962;75:46–54.

Kirchner JA, Scatliff JH, Dey FL, Shedd DP. The pharynx after laryngectomy. Laryngoscope 1963;73:18–33.

Kothary PM, DeSouza LJ. Swallowing without tongue. Bombay Hosp J 1973;15:58–62.

Lambert JR, Tepperman PS, Jimenez J, Newman A. Cervical spine disease and dysphagia. Am J Gastroenterol 1981;76:35–40.

LaVelle CLB, Proctor DB. Clinical pathology of the oral mucosa. Hagerstown, Md.: Harper & Row, 1978.

Leonard JR, Holt GP, Maran AG. Treatment of vocal cord carcinoma by vertical hemilaryngectomy. Ann Otol Rhinol Laryngol 1972;81:469–78.

Litton WB, Leonard JR. Aspiration after partial laryngectomy: cineradiographic studies. Laryngoscope 1969;75:887–908.

Logemann JA, Bytell DE. Swallowing disorders in three types of head and neck surgical patients. Cancer 1979;44:1095–1105.

Myers EN. The role of total glossectomy in the management of cancer of the oral cavity. Otol Clin North Am 1972;5:343–355.

Schobinger R. Spasm of cricopharyngeus muscle as a cause of dysphagia after total laryngectomy. Arch Otolaryngol 1958;67:271–75.

Schoenrock LD, King AY, Everts EC, Schneider HJ, Shumrick DA. Hemilaryngectomy: deglutition evaluation and rehabilitation. Trans Am Acad Ophthalmol Otolaryngol 1972;76:752–57.

Sessions DG, Zill R, Schwartz SL. Deglutition after conservation surgery for cancer of the larynx and hypopharynx. Otolaryngol Head Neck Surg 1979;87:779–96.

Shedd DP. Rehabilitation problems of head and neck cancer patients. J Surg Oncol 1976;8:11–21.

Staple TW, Ogura JH. Cineradiography of the swallowing mechanism following supraglottic subtotal laryngectomy. Radiology 1966;87:226–30.

Staple TW, Ragsdale EF, Ogura JH. The chest roentgenogram following supraglottic laryngectomy. Am J Roentgenol 1967;100:583–87.

Summers GW. Physiologic problems following ablative surgery of the head and neck. Otolaryngol Clin North Am 1974;7:217–50.

Umerah BC, Mukherjee BK, Ibekur O. Cervical spondylosis and dysphagia. J Laryngol Otol 1981;95:1179–83.

Volin RA. Predicting failure to speak after laryngectomy. Laryngoscope 1980;90:1727–36.

Weaver AW, Fleming SM. Partial laryngectomy: analysis of associated swallowing disorders. Am J Surg 1978;136:486–89.

CHAPTER 4

Evaluation of Swallowing Disorders
Robert M. Miller

A detailed special evaluation of a patient known to have or suspected of having dysphagia involves a number of medical and allied medical disciplines, particularly otolaryngology, gastroenterology, and neurology; however, it is not meant to take the place of any other consultation. The examination is intended to evaluate factors that relate to swallowing function (Table 4.1), not to be diagnostic of the underlying disease, although it may either obviate or clarify the need for other studies.

The word dysphagia, according to *Dorland's Illustrated Medical Dictionary,* is derived from the Greek *phagein,* meaning to eat. Conditions that could impair eating are numerous and diverse. Even considering the more limited definition of dysphagia such as "difficulty in swallowing," the complexity involved in special evaluations of patients with such complaints can be appreciated.

The dysphagia examination should be considered a team evaluation, as no one discipline can assess in detail all phases of swallowing. Without attempting to enumerate all of the disciplines that might contribute to a comprehensive special dysphagia examination, and recognizing that responsibilities and expertise will vary from setting to setting, an outline of the relevant systems to be assessed is in order and is presented in Table 4.1.

Disorders of swallowing may be found in diverse patient populations, for example, following acute neurologic events and surgery of the head and neck. Dysphagia is also a manifestation of many subacute progressive neurologic diseases, and may be an isolated symptom found in otherwise stable elderly patients. The special examination for dysphagia will need to be modified and adapted to fit the clinical setting and patient population. The procedures outlined within the chapter, therefore, should be viewed as general guidelines rather than a cookbook approach for examining the dysphagic patient.

Table 4.1.   Comprehensive Evaluation for Dysphagia.

Factors Influencing Swallowing	Methods of Assessment
Oral phase	
Mental status, judgment	Screen orientation, language, visual-motor perception, and memory
Muscles of facial expression	Examine for symmetry at rest and during movement
Muscles of mastication	Palpate and gently resist movement
Mucous membranes	Inspect
Dentition	Inspect
Lingual muscles	Inspect at rest and on protrusion; resist movement
Orofacial sensation	Subjective; identify stimulus qualities
Pharyngeal phase	
Palatopharyngeal closure	Observe at rest and during phonation; stimulate gag reflex
Pharyngeal constriction	Stimulate gag; motion radiography
Extrinsic laryngeal muscles	Palpate larynx during swallow
Intrinsic laryngeal muscles	Indirect laryngeal inspection
Cricopharyngeus muscle	Motion radiography
Esophageal phase	
Morphology of the esophagus	Motion radiography and endoscopy
Esophageal motility	Manometry and cineradiography
Gastroesophageal sphincter function, hiatal hernia, and reflux	Manometry, cineradiography, gastroesophageal scintiscanning, acid perfusion, pH monitoring, endoscopy, and biopsy

WARNING SIGNS

There are several warning signs that should alert health professionals to the likelihood of dysphagia. For example, the presence of a confused mental state or dysarthric speech in a patient with neurologic disease should be cause for special attention to the eating process. Since eating requires some degree of vigilance and planning, patients who exhibit poor judgment, perceptual impairments, or motor planning disorders following any form of brain damage are at risk for swallowing catastrophe. Similarly, dysarthric speech characterized by slow, labored, or slurred articulation, nasal air emission, and hoarse or breathy voice are manifestations of the inherent weakness of muscles common to both speaking and swallowing. An additional symptom suggestive of dysphagia is excessive drooling (sialorrhea), which is often due to motor and/or sensory impairments of the swallowing mechanism. Frequent episodes of coughing and choking on food and sputum should be considered as warning signs for dysphagia. Prolongation of meals, unexplained weight loss, effortful chewing, or difficulty in the oral preparation of a bolus may all signify swallowing difficulty.

A patient's complaint of pain or obstruction during swallowing should be taken seriously as a warning for dysphagia. A clinical finding on indirect laryngeal examination of the pooling sign or accumulation of food debris in the vallecula or pyriform sinuses suggests that the swallowing mechanism has failed completely to clear the bolus from the pharynx into the esophagus. Excessive pooling and the potential for tracheal aspiration may be appreciated on radiographic study of swallows by video or cineradiography.

THE EVALUATION

It is helpful when beginning an examination for dysphagia to have a procedural outline or worksheet available. This will help to ensure that important data will not be overlooked during the assessment.

Subjective Complaints

The history begins with information regarding the present complaint. Frequently, the subjective description of the problem will give the examiner significant clues regarding its cause. In many instances, however, history will not be attainable from the patient as swallowing problems are frequently associated with altered mental states and/or severely impaired speech. In these instances, information may come from a professional observer, health care attendant, family member, or medical records. Specific questions should address such issues as the duration of the problem, the frequency of swallowing difficulty, intermittent versus constant presence, and factors and circumstances that exacerbate or alleviate the problem.

It is particularly important to determine the relative influence of solid, semisolid, and liquid foods on swallowing. In general, patients who suffer from neurologic conditions that weaken or result in dyscoordination of the swallowing mechanism will complain that liquids are more likely to cause choking than solids or semisolids (Linden and Siebens, 1983). Since fluids will naturally spread as they move from the mouth through the pharynx into the esophagus, they require more precise channeling than solids, and therefore are more difficult for weak or uncoordinated motor mechanisms to control. Patients suffering from obstructive conditions such as strictures, tumors, or webs are more likely to complain about solid food sticking or lodging in the throat or esophagus. Although the correlation between the cause of the swallowing difficulty and consistency of the bolus is probably high, caution is recommended to avoid being misled.

In detailing the history, specific questions should be asked that address symptoms frequently associated with dysphagia.

Obstruction

Although most people associate subjective descriptions of obstruction with tumors, strictures, webs, and diverticula, it is also a frequent complaint in patients with neurologic conditions that result in muscle weakness and/or incoordination. The patient should be asked if food sticks, and then directed to point to the level at which they sense the obstruction. Patients with cricopharyngeal dysfunction and those with a pharyngoesophageal (Zenker's) diverticulum usually describe the hang-up at the level of the thyroid cartilage (Jordan, 1977). Those with pooling in the vallecula or pyriform sinuses may also point to an area adjacent to the larynx as the site of obstruction. It should be noted, however, that the area in which the obstruction is sensed by the patient does not always correspond with the site of actual narrowing or blockage as this is demonstrated by radiography.

Nasal Regurgitation

Patients should be asked about episodes of nasopharyngeal regurgitation, that is, liquid or firm food moving up into the nasal cavity rather than down toward the esophagus. An occasional nasal penetration occurring in association with coughing is probably not significant. Frequent episodes of nasal regurgitation suggest some malfunction of the palatal and upper pharyngeal mechanism.

Mouth Odor

Foul mouth odors may be associated with a variety of conditions, including hygiene problems, oral retention of food, dental or periodontal disease, and oral-mucosal lesions which result in necrotic changes. An additional source for mouth odor is Zenker's pharyngoesophageal diverticulum. In these cases, food trapped in the sac can putrify and emit a foul odor. These patients may also describe episodes in which food returns to the mouth, sometimes hours after a meal.

Aspiration

The patient with complaints regarding swallowing should be questioned about episodes of aspiration in which food or liquid tends to go into the windpipe. Coughing or choking frequently while eating is another manifestation of aspiration. Although sensations of aspiration can occur with a variety of conditions, it is probably most common in neuromuscular disorders of swallowing.

Gastroesophageal Reflux

Gastroesophageal reflux is usually identified by patients as a sensation of heartburn. Severe or persistent cases of gastroesophageal reflux may lead to esophageal mucosal irritation, esophageal muscle and sphincter dysfunction, laryngeal mucosal ulceration, and/or aspiration of stomach contents, the latter particularly during sleep.

It should be recognized that reflux is a very common event. The potential for symptomatic gastroesophageal reflux is probably greatest in patients with a hiatal hernia, a condition that is present in about 67 percent of persons over 60 years of age (Straus, 1979). Esophagitis, esophageal ulcer, and esophageal stricture are potential complications of reflux.

Speech and Voice

Since speech and swallowing are dependent on certain common neurologic, muscular, and anatomic factors, changes in speech or voice may parallel the development of swallowing difficulties. Patients should be asked if their speech has changed in any way, for example, hoarseness or temporary loss of voice. A change in articulatory coordination or precision, interpreted by the patient as slurring or clumsy speech, usually reflects neurologic impairment. An isolated voice change may be the consequence of neurologic, neoplastic, or inflammatory disorders.

Pain

Odynophagia, or pain on swallowing, is rarely associated with dysphagia of central nervous system origin. It is more commonly related to infections, neoplasms, or mechanical obstructions in the pharyngeal region. Pain may be a manifestation of an esophageal motor disorder. Esophageal pain is usually perceived substernally, with radiation into the back, jaw, neck, or down the left arm. It may be clinically indistinguishable from the pain of coronary artery disease (Pope, 1977).

Weight Loss

The symptom of weight loss may be related directly to impaired nutritional intake reflecting an underlying disease process. Reported changes in weight is a clinician's yardstick by which progressive dysphagia can be charted and is a means of assessing the effectiveness of a feeding management plan.

Pneumonia

Evidence of recurrent aspiration pneumonia may be associated with neuromuscular incoordination or weakness of the swallowing mechanism. It can result from a patient's inability to protect the airway due to selective muscle paralysis. Paralysis of the vocal cords is particularly significant. Recurrent pneumonia also can be found in patients who have mechanical obstructions of the deglutitory tract or severe gastroesophageal pharyngeal-tracheal reflux. The occurrence of aspiration pneumonia is grossly related to the severity of dysphagia.

Previous Medical History

Information relevant to a patient's swallowing and nutritional status can often be obtained from the general health history. For example, special attention should be paid to neurologic history; cerebrovascular accidents, head trauma, central nervous system infections, and demyelinating diseases are particularly significant in pertinence to dysphagia. All prior surgery should be noted, particularly procedures involving the head and neck or gastrointestinal tract. The patient's psychologic health should be reviewed in search of aspects affecting appetite or food preference.

Medications

Several medications influence swallowing. A list should be compiled of all medications currently prescribed and those that had been taken regularly in the past. Sedative drugs or those that cause disorientation and confusion can have a significant influence upon swallow particularly in brain-damaged patients. For example, slightly toxic doses of some anticonvulsants can add to the confusion of patients with brain trauma and cause decompensation of a previously marginal swallowing mechanism. Medications that potentially weaken muscles, such as some prescribed to reduce spasticity, may exacerbate existing swallowing problems. It is known that some moisture must be present in the mouth in order to elicit a swallow reflex; therefore medications with an action or side effect of diminishing secretions and, thus, drying of the oral, nasal, and pharyngeal mucosae can adversely influence swallowing by delaying initiation of this reflex. Many antipsychotic drugs can lead to extrapyramidal symptoms such as dystonia, motor restlessness, pseudo-parkinsonism, and tardive dyskinesia. Persistent tardive dyskinesia usually causes rhythmic, involuntary movements of the face, jaw, and tongue, each of which may interfere with the initiation and control of chewing and swallowing.

Certain over-the-counter medications and prescribed topical anesthetics used to relieve a sore throat or ticking cough have the potential of impairing swallowing. Some denture powders also contain topical anesthetics that could disturb oral and pharyngeal sensation.

In general, drugs appear to have very little effect upon the function of the esophagus and are not known to cause motor disorders of the esophagus (Christensen, 1976). Moss and Green (1982), however, reported a case of confirmed esophageal dystonia associated with the neuroleptic molindone hydrochloride (Moban).

Physical Examination

In most cases, the description of the problem and background data will dictate the appropriate course to follow in the physical examination. The detailed examination that follows may be used in part or in total, as the case requires. Since dysphagia is almost never functional, patients with swallowing complaints should be examined thoroughly.

The purpose of this examination for the clinical assessment of swallowing is to: (1) establish a possible cause of dysphagia; (2) assess the patient's ability to protect the airway; (3) determine the practicality of oral feeding and/or recommend alternative methods for nutritional management; (4) determine the need for additional diagnostic tests or studies; and (5) establish baseline clinical data that can be used to chart changes in feeding function of patients with progressively deteriorating diseases.

Mental Status

The examination should begin with some assessment of the patient's mental status and ability to cooperate. This is especially true when dealing with patients with known or suspected central nervous system lesions contributing to dysphagia. Larsen (1981) described the problems experienced by patients with left or right brain damage. With right-sided hemiplegia with aphasia, for example, patients may become overwhelmed or confused while attempting to eat in the circumstance of other individuals engaging in conversation. Because of muscle spasticity in combination with the language disorder of aphasia, these patients are at risk for aspiration when trying to combine eating with speaking.

Conversely, Larsen describes right-brain-damaged patients as having problems with the praxis of eating; that is, they are disturbed in organizing the motor sequence that would allow them to move food from plate to mouth. They are at risk of choking because of problems that relate to judgment, decisions of how much food to take in one bite, and how much to chew. These problems are discussed in more detail in Chapter 5.

A screening psychometric-type test can be used to assess perceptual and language functions to anticipate the type of eating problems that could occur and apply the appropriate rehabilitation procedures (Larsen, 1981). Such a test should include: (1) a series of simple verbal and written commands to assess language comprehension; (2) a task that requires the patient to name common objects or geometric forms to assess simple expressive language; (3) a written task to evaluate the patient's ability to spell several common words or write a phrase from dictation; (4) a verbal problem-solving task requiring the patient to interpret the meaning of a sentence or proverb; and (5) a perceptual-motor copying task in which the patient reproduces forms, such as a square, triangle, and cross.

Weight

Weighing the patient is vital when examination data are to be used for charting changes in progressive disease, and when the clinician must assess the effectiveness of a nutritional management plan. These data also will be useful in leading to an understanding of the severity of a swallowing problem.

Muscles of Facial Expression

Facial muscles should be inspected both at rest and during active movement, comparing movement of the two sides for symmetry. The patient should be asked to make grimacing and puckering movements. When possible, the muscles should be palpated to feel for the weakness. The examiner should look particularly at the patient's ability to seal the lips, having the patient puff out the cheeks and hold the air while manual pressure is applied to the cheeks. Lip closure is important in preventing loss of food anteriorly during the oral phase of swallowing.

Muscles of Mastication

The masseter is the most powerful muscle of mastication. It originates at the zygomatic arch and inserts into the angle of the mandible. The temporalis, which serves to adjust the jaw up, forward, or back, originates at the squamous portion of the temporal bone and inserts at the anterior border of the ramus. These two muscles of mastication should be palpated as the patient bites and chews. Gentle resistance can be placed on the mandible to assess the strength of these muscles. Excessive resistance could result in dislocation of the temporomandibular joint. Clinicians recognize that it is almost impossible to swallow with the mouth open.

The grinding action that occurs in chewing is produced by two sets of muscles, the external and internal pterygoids. Their action can be appreciated by instructing the patient to move the mandible from side to side in a rotary action. Again, gentle resistance can be applied to assess the relative strength of these muscles.

Pathologic Reflexes

There are a number of brainstem-level primitive reflexes associated with the chewing and swallowing mechanisms. Normally, these reflexes are inhibited in the adult by higher centers of the brain. Their presence in the adult patient suggests that these higher inhibitory centers are impaired. These pathologic reflexes are seen most commonly in patients with bilateral hemispheric or frontal lobe damage.

The suck reflex may be elicited either by tapping the upper lip with a reflex hammer or by stroking the vermillion border with a tongue blade. Movement of the lips and head in the direction of the stimulus is an abnormal response.

The bite reflex is often elicited in patients with severe neurologic lesions by touching the lips, teeth, or gums with a tongue blade and observing a strong closure of the jaw. This reflex can be particularly troublesome for the examiner, since it may prevent a good oral examination. Attempts to force a jaw open usually result in a stronger bite. The examiner should avoid strong resistance that could result in fracture or dislocation of the mandible. In some patients, spontaneous mouth opening will occur as a stimulus object, such as a spoon or food, is seen approaching the mouth. While the bite reflex can interfere with feeding management, this mouth-opening reflex can be used to aid in the feeding plan.

Oral Mucosa

The intraoral inspection should begin with an assessment of the mucosa. Dentures should be removed prior to this examination. Any pathologic lesions should be noted, and proper diagnostic procedures followed to determine its nature. In many cases this procedure involves consultation with an oral surgeon or otolaryngologist for examination and biopsy.

Particular attention should be paid to the moisture present in the oral cavity. Extreme dryness of the oral and pharyngeal mucosa can virtually prevent voluntary and reflexive swallowing. Thick, tenacious mucus can inhibit swallowing. Any residual oral debris should also be noted.

Dentition

The condition of natural teeth should be noted. Painful teeth can inhibit eating and lead to impaired nutritional states. It should be recognized that dental plates block sensory receptors in the palate and gums that are contributory to the reflex stimulation of chewing. Dental consultation should be considered when dental or other oral disease or abnormality is suspected.

Pharyngeal Palate

The pharyngeal palatine musculature should be evaluated as a unit. In normal swallowing the palate should elevate and the pharynx constrict, allowing a properly masticated bolus to pass over the base of the tongue and enter the hypopharynx without regurgitation into the nasopharynx. Palatopharyngeal constriction should be assessed for symmetry during oral breathing, phonation, and tactual stimulation of the gag reflex. The gag reflex should be elicitable from either side, and the response should be compared on stimulation of each side. The gag is a highly variable reflex even among healthy persons. A diminished gag reflex is probably significant only when found in patients who have evidence of weakened or paralyzed pharyngeal palatine musculature, asymmetric gag reflexes, or other signs of cranial nerve dysfunction. Absence of a gag reflex does not automatically mean that the patient is unable to swallow or protect the airway (Linden and Siebens, 1983).

Tongue

Lingual muscles should be examined for appearance and strength. In the edentulous or highly cooperative patient, palpation of the muscles can be revealing; atrophy, fasciculations, or abnormal movement should be noted. Recognizing that the tongue deviates toward the side of weakness, tongue strength can be grossly assessed by having the patient protrude the tongue. Tongue strength can also be evaluated by instructing the patient to push the tongue firmly against the inner cheek while the examiner resists the movement on each side.

Indirect Laryngoscopy

Indirect laryngoscopy should be performed whenever possible as part of the swallowing examination. A complete examination, as visualized in Figure 4.1, should include inspection of the base of the tongue, vallecula, epiglottis, pyriform sinuses, vocal and vestibular folds, and infraglottic area. Otolar-

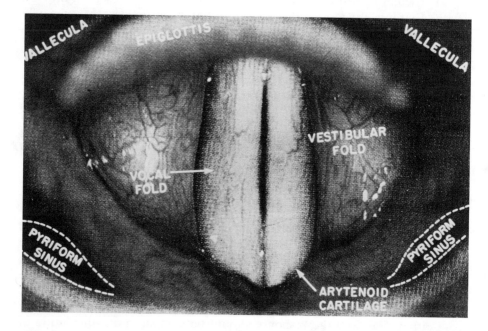

Figure 4.1. Structures visualized on mirror or fiberoptic examination of the larynx.

yngology consultation should be initiated if suspicious mucosal lesions are observed. The vocal cords should be evaluated for function, with observation of symmetry of movement during quiet breathing, forced inhalation, and phonation. Vocal cord function is essential in airway protection during the pharyngeal stage of swallowing and for coughing.

Presence of the pooling sign, detection of food debris, or secretions in the vallecula or pyriform sinuses is an indication that the swallow reflex has been incomplete in clearing the bolus from the pharynx into the esophagus. When pooling is observed adjacent to the aditus of the larynx, the probability of tracheal aspiration is high.

Test Swallows

In normal swallowing a bolus is worked into the oropharynx by muscles of the lips, tongue, and cheek. As the swallow reflex begins, the muscles suspending the larynx contract and draw the larynx up to bury the epiglottis in the base of the tongue. The pharyngeal constrictors strip the bolus toward the cricopharyngeal sphincteric muscle, which opens ahead of the bolus and allows it to pass into the esophagus. An examiner can appreciate the moment of swallowing by placing a finger on the thyroid notch between the hyoid bone and the larynx and feel the larynx move up and forward during the swallow reflex. If the muscles are weak or the reflexes inadequate, the examiner's finger may fail to be deflected by elevation of the larynx. In this case, the cricopharyngeus may fail to open properly and the epiglottis will not be adequately buried in the base of the tongue, thus leaving the airway unprotected.

On palpation of the laryngeal cartilages in some elderly patients, the larynx will be noted in an abnormally low position. This condition, laryngoptosis, may contribute to inadequate airway protection during swallowing.

Testing the adequacy of a swallow brings a certain degree of risk for aspiration. Coughing itself is not an indication that the patient is experiencing tracheal aspiration. In fact, the cough reflex is the final protective mechanism to prevent aspiration. The presence of an adequate cough reflex is necessary before an oral nutritional management program can be established. If the patient has lost or has an inadequate cough reflex, even test swallows with most foods and liquids are unsafe. Although a voluntary cough should be elicited and judged, the examiner should recognize that voluntary and reflexive coughs can be quite different in quality and effectiveness. Patients with cortical brain damage are frequently unable voluntarily to organize motor behaviors necessary to produce a good cough, but their reflexive cough is intact. Conversely, there are rare cases in which patients can voluntarily cough, but because of an impaired sensorimotor complex, the reflexive cough is lost. Measurement of vital capacity is sometimes a helpful adjunct in predicting the effectiveness of a cough reflex.

Initially, it is advisable to use a substance that is relatively safe if partially aspirated, and to be absolutely certain that the patient is able to cough to protect the airway in case of aspiration. A spoonful of crushed ice is relatively safe and will provide a good medium for eliciting the chewing reflex because of its texture and cold stimulation to the receptors in the gums. The examiner should observe the chewing action and feel for laryngeal elevation to indicate that a swallow has occurred. Once it is determined that the patient adequately elevates the larynx and there is an adequate protective cough, the examination can proceed to using other substances with different textures and consistencies. During test swallows the examiner should take note of coughing, aspiration, or nasal regurgitation. See Chapter 5 for further discussion.

Some examiners attempt to demonstrate subtle weaknesses of the muscles and protective reflexes by testing swallowing under unfavorable circumstances. For example, it is known that the airway is more protected if a patient swallows with the head and neck flexed. Therefore, placing the patient in a posture with the neck extended and chin up may impair swallow. Patients who can overcome this postural disadvantage are more likely to have an adequate swallow. Similarly, swallowing can be compromised by manually stabilizing the larynx and hyoid bone in order to bring out weakness of the muscles of laryngeal elevation (Figure 4.2).

Swallowing reflexes are subject to fatigue and to warm-up. Test swallows should be performed successively to evaluate for fatiguability when the subjective complaint suggests this possibility. When the initial test swallow is judged to be inadequate due to coughing, additional tests may show improved function. This is particularly true when patients have pooled secretions in the valleculae and pyriform sinuses. They may spill these secretions into the larynx when swallowing is stimulated initially, but improve with swallowing efforts.

Aspiration is difficult to evaluate. If a patient is observed to experience some choking or respiratory distress that is not immediately relieved by coughing, it is probable that some aspiration has taken place. Some examiners listen with a stethoscope placed against the larynx during the swallow and have learned to perceive a characteristic sound of air mixing with liquids that suggests aspiration. Change in a patient's color, gurgling breath sounds, and extreme breathiness, or loss of voice may indicate acute aspiration. Objectively, aspiration can be documented by radiographic studies. During test swallows the examiner should also note nasal regurgitation. This is more common when testing with liquids. Following each swallow, the oral cavity should be inspected for retention of food. Patients with damage to the parietal lobe of the brain and unilateral neglect commonly pocket food on the neglected side.

Test swallows for patients with tracheostoma tubes present distinctive problems. Tracheostoma tubes have a tendency to tether the larynx and trachea, resulting in inefficient laryngeal elevation and tilting (Bonanno, 1971). Sasaki and associates (1977) pointed out that the laryngeal closure reflex is weakened and dyscoordinated when the upper airway is bypassed

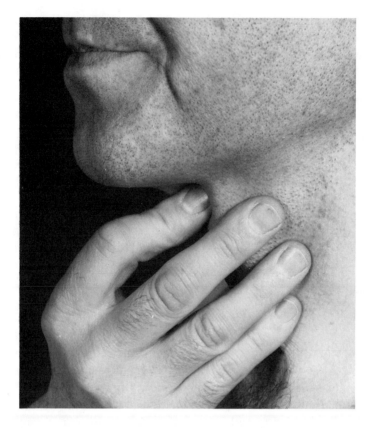

Figure 4.2. Manual stabilization technique of the larynx and hyoid bone.

by tracheostomy. The combination of the tethering effect and impaired protective laryngeal closure reflex leaves the larynx more susceptible to penetration, and the patient is less able to expel the material to prevent tracheal aspiration.

Testing patients who have cuffed tracheostoma swallowing tubes should be done with the cuff deflated. The trachea above the cuff must be suctioned before the cuff is deflated. Before testing swallow, the tracheostoma tube should be plugged for several seconds to assess the patient's ability to breathe through the larynx as well as the voluntary laryngeal cough. As with other patients, laryngeal elevation should be felt during a swallow.

Ice chips provide an adequate stimulus to elicit the initial swallows. Aspiration should be checked by using a stimulus that is dyed with a contrast color that can be detected in the trachea. Methylene blue, 0.5 ml in 30 ml of water, provides an adequate contrast. As the patient drinks approximately 10 ml of colored solution, the examiner observes for evidence of aspiration: in a patient with inadequate swallowing and unprotected airway, the solution may show up immediately in the trachea. The trachea should be suctioned and the contents examined for evidence of the colored solution. Color contrast solutions such as methylene blue tend to coat the entire oropharyngeal mucosa, and it is not unusual to find a very small amount of blue-tinged secretion in the tracheostoma several minutes after a test swallow. This is a very common finding and usually is not associated with inadequate swallowing (Cameron, Reynolds, and Zuidema, 1973).

Greenbaum (1976) suggested a protocol for the decannulation of the patient who has a cuffed tracheostoma tube. The patient is required to drink four ounces of methylene blue-dyed water at intervals of 15 minutes for an hour. The trachea is then thoroughly suctioned and secretions are inspected for evidence of blue coloration. If this test is negative, the cuff is deflated for meals and at other times, with close supervision for 24 hours. Greenbaum added that even though a positive test suggests aspiration, it is not automatically a contraindication to decannulation if the patient demonstrates adequate swallowing during meals with the cuff deflated.

Just as tracheostoma tubes can interfere with the swallow reflex and the protective reflexes in the larynx, nasogastric feeding tubes interfere with normal swallowing by altering sensations in the pharynx and deflecting the bolus. A tube passing transnasally may force the patient to breathe from the mouth, thus drying mucosa and additionally impairing normal reflexes. Some patients may be further decompensated by even a mild degree of dehydration. The examiner must be cognizant of all mechanical and metabolic factors that impede swallowing and the protective reflexes. In some cases, before final decisions can be made to proceed with oral feeding plans, the patient's swallowing should be assessed with tracheostoma and nasogastric tubes removed, the mucosa moist, and the patient adequately nourished and hydrated.

Repeat Indirect Laryngoscopy

After testing a patient's swallow reflex, a repeat indirect examination of the larynx should be performed. Here again, evidence of excessive pooling of debris in the vallecula or pyriform sinuses suggests the swallowing reflex has not completely cleared the bolus from the hypopharynx. Tracheal aspiration might also be appreciated by this repeat examination when the debris is visualized adjacent to the aditus of the larynx or subglottally.

Sensation

Chewing, salivary flow, and swallowing are all reflexes that are, in part, dependent on sensory stimulation. Sensations of hot, cold, pressure, and texture, carried by the trigeminal nerve, are known to stimulate chewing. Taste, which is carried by the facial and glossopharyngeal nerves, plays a role in stimulating salivary flow and, eventually, swallowing (see Chapter 1). If the gag reflex is absent, if the patient drools, if the mucosa is extremely dry, or if food debris is retained in the mouth, some sensory loss involving oral structures may be suspected. Sensory loss alone is rarely the cause of dysphagia.

Many patients can detect and report sensory loss reliably, but in some instances clinicians may wish to test further. For purposes of evaluating functional swallowing, gross touch can be assessed on the face, lips, and buccal mucosa using a cotton swab. Taste may be evaluated by having the patient identify a small sip of juice or the flavors of salt, sour, bitter, and sweet applied to various areas of the tongue with a moistened cotton swab.

Voice and Articulation

The quality of a patient's speech should be assessed as a part of the swallowing evaluation. Speech is an extremely complex, overlearned behavior, and as such, serves as a barometer from which the examiner can assess the status of the neuromuscular system that also serves swallowing. Patients should be asked to sustain a vowel with the examiner noting duration, quality (hoarseness, breathiness, and harshness), pitch, and intensity. Articulation should be assessed for precision and speed. The use of diadochokinetic tasks (forced rapid alternating movements) using consonant-vowel combinations is recommended. Both hypernasal and hyponasal speech qualities should be noted. Hypernasality suggests impaired palatopharyngeal function. Hyponasality implies filling of the nasopharynx or occlusion of nasal passages.

ADDITIONAL STUDIES

To a great extent the physical examination for swallowing is subjective and provides little quantifiable information. It is, however, an indispensable part of the overall evaluation of dysphagia. The practical and functional information often leads to effective management and treatment of conditions that impair the eating process. For many patients the functional evaluation of swallowing is complete once the subjective complaint, history, and peripheral physical findings have been recorded and considered. This is usually the case when they are examined for acute swallowing difficulty following stroke, head trauma, or head and neck surgery. A high percentage of patients with swallowing difficulties of a progressive or chronic nature, especially involving the esophagus, require further evaluation using additional radiologic and other medical studies.

Radiographic Studies

When the findings obtained from the peripheral examination of the swallowing mechanism do not completely explain the symptoms of dysphagia, or the initial evaluation suggests cricopharyngeal, esophageal, or gastro-esophageal junction problems, further work-up is in order. Radiographic studies using high-speed motion pictures or videotaped fluoroscopic swallows are essential for the evaluation of suspected motor disorders of the esophagus. Spot films may be useful to record morphologic changes in the esophagus, but they are not helpful in recording changes in esophageal motility (Stewart, 1981). Ekberg and Nylander (1982b) reported that of 250 consecutive patients with dysphagia studied by cineradiography, 80 percent demonstrated underlying functional disturbances, most of which were not detected by single film studies.

Cineradiography is useful in the evaluation of (1) pharyngeal constriction and the dynamics of airway protection; (2) upper esophageal sphincter function; (3) esophageal motility; (4) lower esophageal sphincter function; (5) morphology of the esophagus; (6) hiatal hernia; and (7) gastroesophageal reflux.

Stewart (1981) outlined a recommended sequence for cineradiographic evaluations. He suggested that the study begin with the patient standing, being examined from both the anteroposterior and lateral projections. This position allows the examiner to assess pharyngeal and upper esophageal sphincter function, particularly with regard to the patient's ability to protect the airway. The erect posture does not provide adequate assessment of esophageal motility. Pope (1977) warned that unless esophageal motility is assessed with the patient supine or in a slightly head-down posture, the cineradiographic study only evaluates the effects of gravity, and esophageal motility will likely be misread as normal.

To study esophageal motility, Stewart (1981) stated that the most convenient patient posture is prone oblique facing the examiner. The patient should take a 7 to 10 cc bolus of barium through a straw. The patient should be instructed to swallow only once, because the esophageal peristaltic wave can be interrupted by additional swallows. An adequate study requires at least three separate swallows. Patients who are unable to take the barium through a straw can have the bolus injected by a syringe. For those who are unable to channel the bolus into the esophagus or who cannot cooperate, a nasoesophageal tube can be inserted for the purpose of injecting a bolus into the upper esophagus. This technique will generally elicit a secondary peristaltic wave and allow some assessment of esophageal motility, although it precludes evaluation of the oropharyngeal swallowing mechanism.

When spontaneous gastroesophageal reflux is not observed, Stewart (1981) recommended the use of provocative techniques to elicit reflux. These techniques include placing the patient in the Trendelenburg position, leg raising, performing Valsalva maneuvers, turning the patient 360 degrees, and a water-siphon test. When reflux occurs spontaneously or is elicited by provocative techniques, the amount of reflux, its level in the esophagus, and its clearance by secondary peristaltic wave action should be described.

Liquid barium is not entirely satisfactory as a medium for evaluating the presence of mucosal lesions. A bolus such as a marshmallow or bread impregnated with barium is more likely to reveal an area of narrowing. When the bolus is arrested in its descent, attention will be called to this segment. The solid bolus also is helpful in assessing esophageal motility.

Cineradiographic studies can play a role in the evaluation of the oral and pharyngeal stages of swallowing. The examiner should note delays in initiating the passage of barium into the pharynx, misdirection of the bolus into the nasopharynx (Figure 4.3) or into the laryngeal vestibule, asymmetry of the pyriform sinuses during the swallow, and epiglottic dysfunction (Ekberg and Nylander, 1982a). Cineradiography may be the best tool for assessing upper esophageal sphincter function (Pope, 1977) (Figure 4.4). Dysfunction of the cricopharyngeal muscle, as illustrated in Figure 4.5, was observed in 22 percent of the 250 dysphagic patients studied by Ekberg and

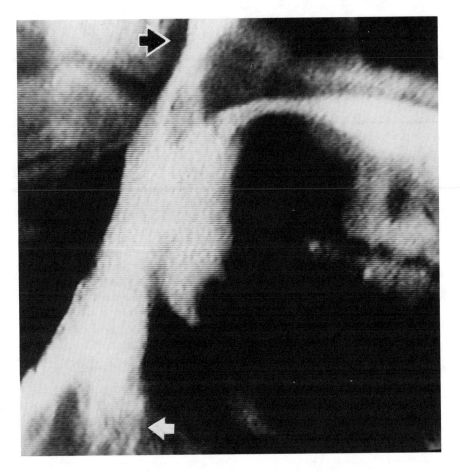

Figure 4.3. Lateral cineradiograph of a patient with contrast medium misdirected into the nasopharynx *(black arrow)* and larynx *(white arrow)*.

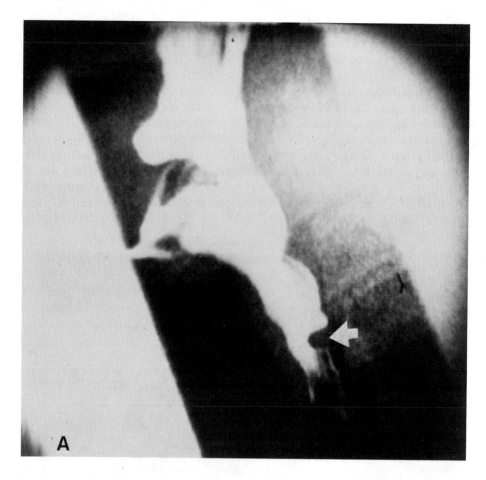

Figure 4.4. Sequential cineradiography of a patient with cricopharyngeal dysfunction. (A) Indentation in the posterior wall of the hypopharynx. (B) A web can be visualized in the upper esophagus *(curved arrow)*. (C) At the completion of the pharyngeal stage of swallowing, contrast medium is retained craniad to the cricopharyngeus. Reprinted with permission of the publisher, from Ekberg and Nylander, *Radiology,* vol. 143, May 1982.

Nylander (1982b). The presence of abnormal pooling in the vallecula and pyriform sinuses, pharyngeal tumors, vertebral osteophytes, and Zenker's diverticula (Figure 4.6) may be revealed through these techniques.

Pope (1977) noted that radiography remains the most available method for evaluating esophageal motor function, but cautioned that the information is not quantifiable and interpretation remains subjective. Diagnoses of esophageal spasm (Figure 4.7) or achalasia of the gastroesophageal sphincter (Figure 4.8), although suspected on cineradiographic study, must be confirmed by other techniques (Hellemans et al., 1981).

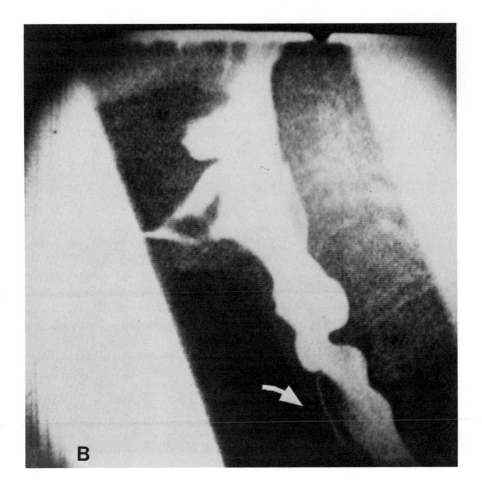

Figure 4.4.   *(continued)*

Manometry

Intraluminal esophageal manometry is a method of quantifying the velocity of peristalsis and the force of esophageal contractions (Dodds, 1976). It is the best means of assessing sphincteric relaxation, particularly in the lower esophageal segment (Pope, 1977). Manometry uses pressure transducers spaced within a catheter that can be passed into the esophagus, allowing simultaneous measurement of pressures at various levels of the esophagus (Figure 4.9). Although cricopharyngeal dysfunction is not always substantiated by manometry, this procedure is particularly useful in diagnosing conditions such as achalasia, diffuse spasms of the esophagus, aperistalsis, and other unclassified motor disorders of the esophagus (Pope, 1977).

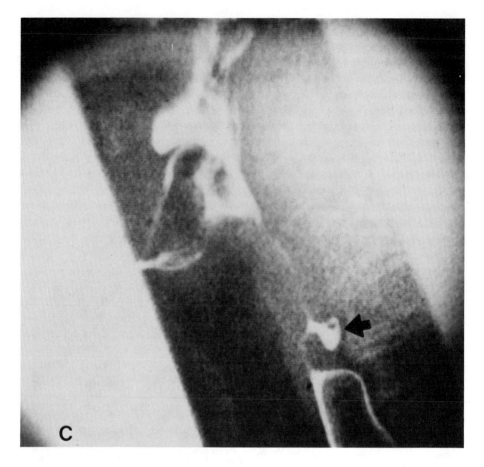

Figure 4.4.   *(continued)*

Reflux Tests

Although it is common for asymptomatic patients to experience occasional esophageal reflux during the day, severe and frequent reflux may lead to distressing symptoms. The most common of these is heartburn, or substernal chest pain. Aspiration can be a complication of reflux, as can esophagitis. Histologic changes are commonly found in symptomatic patients. Increased cricopharyngeal pressure has been found in patients with symptomatic reflux. This potential complication is thought to be a compensation to help prevent aspiration (Hutcheon and Hendrix, 1977). Dysphagia may be a consequence of reflux in patients with esophageal spasm or peptic stricture.

Tests for reflux, in addition to the radiologic studies described, may include gastroesophageal scintiscanning, the acid perfusion test, and the esophageal pH-monitoring acid reflux test.

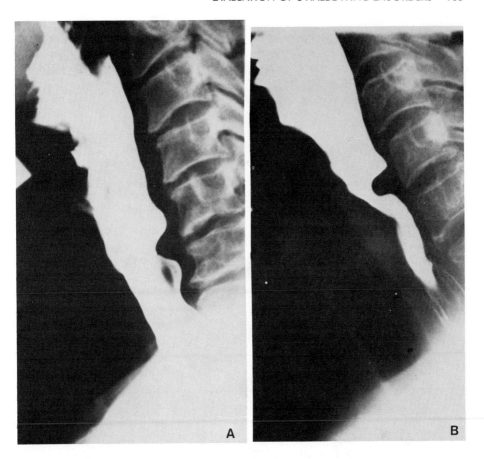

Figure 4.5. Indentation of the cricopharyngeal muscle revealed by cineradiography may be found in varying degrees. (A) Indentation of 25 to 50 percent of the sagittal diameter is seen. (B) Indentation of more than 50 percent of the diameter of the esophagus. Reprinted with permission of the publisher, from Ekberg and Nylander, *Radiology,* vol. 143, May 1982.

Gastroesophageal scintiscanning has been described as a reliable means of detecting and quantifying esophageal reflux (Fisher et al., 1976). A radionuclide preparation is instilled into the stomach by catheter and the patient's thorax is scintiscanned for evidence of radioactive material in the esophagus. Any radioactivity detected cephalad to the lower esophageal sphincter represents esophageal reflux.

An acid perfusion test has been developed to aid in differentiation of painful esophageal disorders due to reflux from cardiovascular chest pain (Bennett and Atkinson, 1966; Hutcheon and Hendrix, 1977). By perfusing saline solution alternately with decinormal hydrochloric acid through a nasogastric tube placed in the esophagus, the test attempts to reproduce the

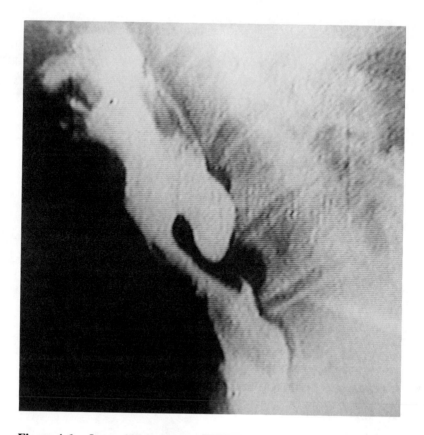

Figure 4.6. Lateral cineradiograph shows a posterior hypopharyngeal pouch that is dilated at the height of the pharyngeal stage of swallowing. A Zenker's diverticulum can be diagnosed on cineradiography, but cannot be distinguished from a pseudodiverticulum on a single radiograph.

patient's typical symptoms. When pain is produced by acid perfusion but not with saline, the test is considered positive.

Another acid reflux test involves placing a pH probe 5 cm above the gastroesophageal junction and recording changes in esophageal pH. The recordings are taken for about 15 minutes while the patient performs provocative maneuvers to increase intra-abdominal pressure. According to Hutcheon and Hendrix (1977), this test discriminates well between symptomatic patients and controls. Twenty-four-hour monitoring of esophageal pH is more cumbersome and therefore less clinically valuable. Such monitoring has shown that both symptomatic patients and controls have reflux during the day, but it occurs in symptomatic patients more frequently and for longer periods at night.

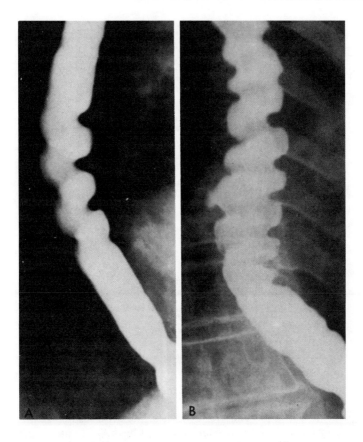

Figure 4.7. (A) Localized midesophageal spasm.
(B) More diffuse esophageal spasm. Reprinted with per-
mission of the publisher, from Stewart, *Medical Clinics of
North America,* vol. 65, 1981.

Endoscopy

For conditions of dysphagia that cannot adequately be explained on the basis
of the peripheral physical examination, radiography, and manometry, en-
doesophagoscopy may be indicated. Although not recommended as a primary method for evaluating motor dysfunction in the esophagus, it is useful
for diagnosing local lesions, particularly to rule out cancer mimicking the
symptoms of achalasia (Pope, 1977). Endoscopy is helpful in diagnosing
complications due to reflux, with biopsy in 95 percent of symptomatic patients
showing both hyperplasia and elongation of vascular papillae (Hutcheon and
Hendrix, 1977).

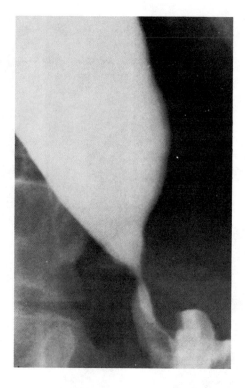

Figure 4.8. In a patient with achalasia, the lower esophageal sphincter is narrowed and seen as a "bird beak." The atonic esophagus above is dilated with barium. Reprinted with permission of the publisher, from Stewart, *Medical Clinics of North America,* vol. 65, 1981.

SUMMARY

No one practitioner can be expected to gather the pertinent historical information, conduct the clinical physical examination, and administer and interpret all of the specialized tests for dysphagia and related problems. The patient with dysphagia deserves a thorough evaluation that can be coordinated by health professionals who are familiar with all aspects of the deglutitory process and the details of a thorough evaluation. Ideally, a team of clinicians can work together to provide the diagnostic tests and functional information needed to assist patients with swallowing problems.

The discussion of the special examination of the patient with dysphagia is an overview of the most common evaluation techniques available. The diagnostic information obtained is useful when it is integrated with the general medical examination, including laboratory data. Functional information, however, should be sufficient to plan for appropriate feeding management,

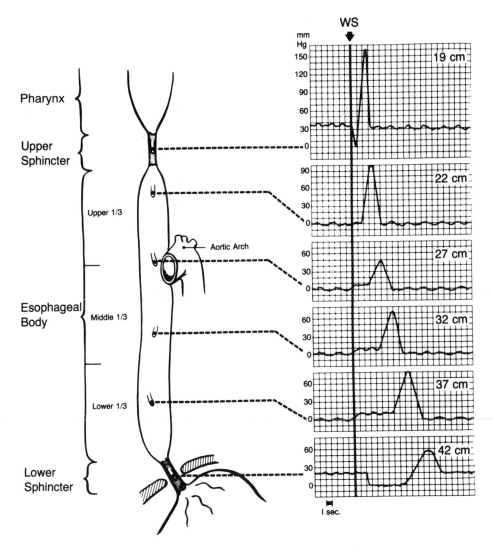

Figure 4.9. Schematic representation of esophageal pressures obtained from intraluminal manometry at rest and after a wet swallow. Reprinted by permission of the publisher, from Dodds, *Archives of Internal Medicine,* vol. 136, no. 5, May 1976, 515–23. © 1976, American Medical Association.

swallowing rehabilitation, or alternative approaches to nutritional management.

REFERENCES

Bennett JR, Atkinson M. The differentiation between oesophageal and cardiac pain. Lancet 1966;2:1123–27.

Bonanno PC. Swallowing dysfunction after tracheostomy. Ann Surg 1971;174:29–33.

Cameron JL, Reynolds J, Zuidema GD. Aspiration in patients with tracheostomies. Surg Gynecol Obstet 1973;136:68–70.

Christensen J. Effects of drugs on esophageal motility. Arch Intern Med 1976;136(5):532–37.

Dodds WJ. Instrumentation and methods for intraluminal esophageal manometry. Arch Intern Med 1976;136:515–23.

Ekberg O, Nylander G. Cineradiography of the pharyngeal stage of deglutition in 150 individuals without dysphagia. Br J Radiol 1982a;55:253–57.

Ekberg O, Nylander G. Cineradiography of the pharyngeal stage of deglutition in 250 patients with dysphagia. Br J Radiol 1982b;55:258–62.

Ekberg O, Nylander G. Dysfunction of the cricopharyngeus muscle: a cineradiographic study of patients with dysphagia. Radiology 1982;143:481–6.

Fisher RS, Malmud LS, Roberts GS, Lobis IF. Gastroesophageal (GE) scintiscanning to detect and quantitate GE reflux. Gastroenterology 1976;70(3):301–8.

Greenbaum DM. Decannulation of the tracheostomized patient. Heart Lung 1976;5(1):119–23.

Hellemans J, Agg HO, Pelemans W, Vantrappen G. Pharyngoesophageal swallowing disorders and the pharyngoesophageal sphincter. Med Clin North Am 1981;65(6):1149–71.

Hutcheon DF, Hendrix TR. Esophageal reflux: diagnosis and therapy. Postgrad Med 1977;61(2):131–37.

Jordan PH. Dysphagia and esophageal diverticula. Postgrad Med 1977;61(2):155–61.

Larsen GL. Chewing and swallowing. In: Martin N, Holt N, Hicks DJ, eds. Comprehensive rehabilitation nursing. New York: McGraw-Hill, 1981;174–85.

Linden P, Siebens AA. Dysphagia: predicting laryngeal penetration. Arch Phys Med Rehabil 1983;64:281–4.

Moss HB, Green A. Neuroleptic-associated dysphagia confirmed by esophageal manometry. Am J Psychiatry 1982;139(4):515–16.

Pope CE. Motor disorders of the esophagus. Postgrad Med 1977;61(2):118–25.

Sasaki CT, Suzuki M, Horiuchi M, Kirchner JA. The effect of tracheostomy on the laryngeal closure reflex. Laryngoscope 1977;87(9, part 1):1428–33.

Stewart ET. Radiographic evaluation of the esophagus and its motor disorders. Med Clin North Am 1981;65(6):1173–94.

Straus B. Disorders of the digestive system. In: Rossman I, ed. Clinical geriatrics. 2d ed. Philadelphia: J B Lippincott 1979;266–89.

PART II

Clinical Management of Swallowing Disorders

CHAPTER 5

General Treatment of Neurologic Swallowing Disorders

Robert M. Miller and Michael E. Groher

An early and accurate diagnosis and evaluation of patients suspected of having dysphagia secondary to neurologic disease is essential for the design of safe and effective treatment. The neurogenic causes for dysphagia are numerous (see Chapter 2) and it is important that the dysphagia specialist become familiar with the clinical pathologic mechanisms of certain disease processes. This should include a thorough understanding of effects on the neuromuscular system, clinical course and expected prognosis, changes that medical or surgical intervention might bring, and potential effects on the patient's learning skills. The interaction of these factors should determine the proper approach to management.

The most challenging aspect of neurologically based swallowing disorders is that patients with similar pathologic processes develop swallowing disorders which differ in severity and in schedule. For instance, all patients with amyotrophic lateral sclerosis (ALS) will not develop similar patterns of dysphagia and therefore require identical therapy. In some ALS patients, dysphagia is a significant problem at first diagnosis. In others it is not evident until the later stages of the disease, and even then, its clinical manifestations may differ among individuals. Even though dysphagia with significant aspiration may be part of a well-known set of clinical signs for a particular neurologic disease, it may not manifest itself in an identical manner, and may be demonstrated at unpredictable times. Even when dysphagia becomes apparent, patients with identical causative conditions require different treatment approaches due to disease severity, previous medical history, willingness to cooperate and/or learn, and present state of health. Successful management is dependent on an awareness of such disparities.

These introductory comments alert the reader to the fact that the treatment concepts presented in this chapter should not be generalized. The approaches described are to be used only as guidelines for treatment. Overgeneralization may result in inflexibility in dealing with patients who require a great deal of adaptation of treatment. Unfortunately, each patient will not benefit from our suggestions; however, with continued investigation and the application of individualized clinical problem solving, those with neurogenic dysphagia can be managed effectively. Specific neurofacilitative approaches to deglutition management that often are used as precursors to oral intake are covered in Chapter 6.

TREATMENT OF DYSPHAGIA PARALYTICA

Diseases that affect the lower motoneurons of the brainstem or their peripheral connections to the swallowing muscles may render the musculature needed for swallow either weak or paretic. There may be several disorders of cranial innervation so that the ability to swallow is incapacitated. Facial and/or hypoglossal nerve involvement may be present. The cough reflex, which is mediated by the ninth and tenth cranial nerves, may be so impaired that the patient is unable to expel accumulated secretions or a bolus that has penetrated the larynx. Cineradiography may demonstrate failure of the cricopharyngeus muscle to relax, thus incapacitating pharyngeal swallow. The principal causes of dysphagia secondary to lower motoneuron involvement are discussed in Chapter 2.

Because the respiratory centers are located in the brainstem, and because of patients' failure adequately to control their own secretions, those with dysphagia paralytica may require a tracheostoma. Their critical medical condition in the acute stages often requires intravenous and subsequent nasogastric tube, or bypass feeding to support life.

Although one of the goals of a swallowing management program is to avoid the prolonged use of nasogastric tube feedings, these are particularly important in the initial stages of medical management because they supply the nutrients that may eventually give the patient the strength to begin receiving nutrition orally. As metabolic balance is achieved, critical protective reflexes may return and a swallowing treatment plan can be implemented.

Such a feeding program should not begin until the physician feels the patient's acute medical status warrants it. The swallowing evaluation must demonstrate that the patient has an adequate protective and productive cough reflex and can elevate the larynx during a swallow (see Chapter 4). Ideally, the cannula will be removed, as the tracheostoma tube may interfere with normal laryngeal elevation and cricopharyngeal relaxation (Bonanno, 1971).

Swallowing management and treatment of patients with dysphagia paralytica is based on five major concepts: (1) establish an effective means of communication; (2) use a safe and stimulating diet in an effort to trigger a weak reflex; (3) capitalize on intact voluntary cortical drive to facilitate swallowing; (4) strengthen weakened oral and pharyngeal musculature; and (5) attempt surgical intervention.

Communication

Before consideration can be given to diet and muscle strengthening exercises, the clinician's work will be greatly facilitated if a viable communication system is established between patient and staff. Due to the weakened articulatory muscles, patients with dysphagia paralytica often cannot produce intelligible speech even though their mental abilities with respect to language remain intact. Electronic communication aids, silent spokesman boards (Figure 5.1), and yes/no question strategies are all commonly employed modes of communication that aid in the patient's treatment. It is very beneficial to the clinician if the patient can express difficulties and successes that occur during swallowing remediation.

Diet

If the swallow reflex is absent or very weak, patients with brainstem pathology need maximal dietary stimulus to give the reflex the best chance to respond. Rather than recommending the traditional pureed foods, a diet that enhances the sensations of taste, temperature, texture, and pressure is recommended. Purees appeal to none of these, and in fact, they might be more difficult to swallow because of their bland taste, unappealing appearance, lack of temperature and texture, and minimal pressure requirements for chewing (Figure 5.2). Purees are difficult to control in the oral cavity when the musculature is weakened, and the patient with lower motoneuron weakness finds it difficult to form the necessary bolus to trigger a swallow. For the same reason, fluids often are harder to control than semisolids. Some patients with dysphagia paralytica who also have accompanying cricopharyngeal dysfunction may find that if the reflex is elicited, softer foods and liquids pass into the esophagus more easily, while solids are obstructed at this level due to failure of the sphincter to relax or because of premature sphincter closure.

In general, patients with lower motoneuron dysphagia should avoid foods such as applesauce that falls apart as it passes through the pharynx, fresh white bread or bananas that are sticky and tend to hang up, and chocolate or ice cream that increases heavy mucus retention, which can in itself become an interference.

Muscle Strengthening

If patients demonstrate that they are unable to take liquids safely, and solids fail to reach the esophagus, they perhaps can be taught to swallow a naso-

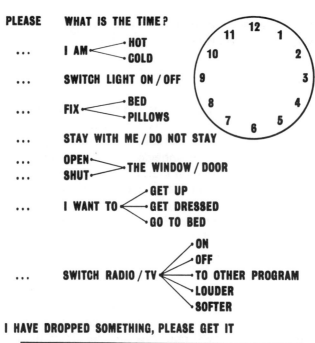

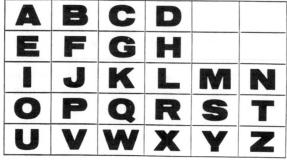

Figure 5.1. Example of a "silent spokesman" communicator. The patient is able to communicate by pointing to specific needs or complaints.

gastric feeding tube orally (Figure 5.3). Because the gag reflex already is diminished or absent, the patient may find this easy to do. Stimulation of the tongue and pharyngeal muscle bundles by the tube during oral passage may activate contraction of weakened muscles. By reciprocal action, enhancement of contraction of the inferior constrictor allows the cricopharyngeus to relax. The patient will not only be able to self-administer nutrition, but at the same time will receive the added benefit of strengthening the muscles needed for swallowing with an easily retrievable bolus. Intermittent passage of the tube allows the patient to receive nutrition, water, and med-

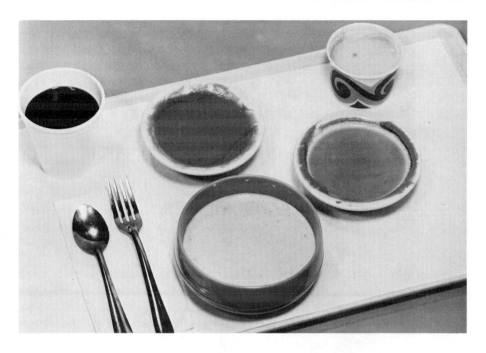

Figure 5.2.   Typical pureed food consisting of strained vegetables, thinned apple-sauce, soup, and coffee. All items are liquid and appear unappetizing in addition to their bland flavoring.

ication and avoids the constant irritation of a nasogastric tube. With recovery, sensation and active reflexes in the pharynx may return. If the patient reports nausea during orogastric tube passage or while the tube is in place, the procedure should be discontinued until the cause is determined. Emesis must be avoided because of the potential for aspiration of stomach contents.

Passage of an oral tube can be used as an exercise for swallowing in which the patient uses the tongue and facial muscles to move the tube back and attempts to elevate the larynx. In patients with paralysis of swallowing due to progressive degenerative neurologic diseases such as ALS or exacerbation of myasthenia gravis, exercises for strengthening are contraindicated. For them, the feeding tube can be passively inserted and used as a tool for nutritional management.

Intellectual Controls

Since most of the patients with dysphagia paralytica retain intellectual functions and some voluntary (upper motoneuron) control of the swallowing musculature, this can be used to advantage during feeding. Once the treat-

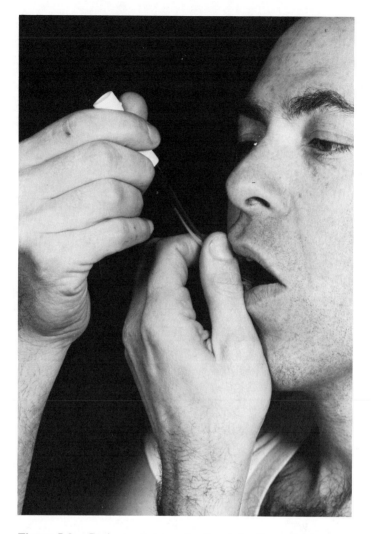

Figure 5.3.   Patient passing a feeding tube through his
mouth. This serves as a convenient way to take nutrition and
helps to exercise weakened oral and pharyngeal musculature.

ment plan has advanced to the point of using food and liquid to stimulate
swallowing, the patient's attention can be focused on fully appreciating the
taste, feel, and temperature of the bolus. Once the bolus has moved posteriorly in the oral cavity, the patient should concentrate on swallowing.
This often will trigger a reflex when the bolus alone fails to activate the
weakened muscles (Larsen, 1976). Some patients can be taught to hold a
full breath consciously during each swallow and produce a gentle voluntary

cough on completion of the swallow. This procedure may assist in protecting the airway.

Surgical Alternatives

At times it is appropriate to consider surgical intervention either to improve the chances of the patient swallowing and protecting the airway, or to provide an alternative route by which the patient can receive food and water. If radiography demonstrates that the cricopharyngeus has failed to relax, the patient may be a candidate for a myotomy of this sphincter. If the problem is unilateral vocal cord paralysis and associated ineffectiveness of cough, the patient may be considered for Teflon injection of the paralyzed cord to improve glottic closure and thereby enhance the strength of the cough. Following these procedures, the patient may be able to continue successfully with oral intake.

It is important to remember that many patients with brainstem pathology such as those with end-stage demyelinating diseases will not improve or show increased strength in the swallowing musculature. As a consequence, their nutritional intake will not be through the oral route and a surgical alternative must be considered. In most cases we favor the feeding esophagostomy (English, Morfit, and Ratzer, 1970) over the gastrostomy because the patient can sit in an upright position while eating, which aids in proper digestion; the tube can be removed between feedings, which is to the patient's psychologic advantage; skin care is minimal; and the procedure is easily reversible should the patient's neurologic status improve.

If a patient is incapable of protecting the airway from aspiration, and recurrent aspiration pneumonia is a problem, considerations for surgery might include laryngeal closure (Montgomery, 1975), tracheoesophageal anastomosis (Lindemann, 1975), or even laryngectomy (Smith et al., 1965). With each of these procedures voice is sacrificed, but aspiration is eliminated. Alternative forms of communication then become a primary consideration. (See Chapter 10 for a full discussion of surgical issues and procedures.)

TREATMENT OF PSEUDOBULBAR DYSPHAGIA

Of the patients with neurologic disease whom we have examined for dysphagia, the majority have pseudobulbar dysphagia. Typically, this is the result of bilateral upper motoneuron involvement. The patient frequently has had bilateral capsular infarctions, the first of which may cause transitory dysphagia, and successive infarcts cause further dysphagia. This is not unusual when we are reminded of the distinctive bilateral representation of the swallowing coordination. Pseudobulbar dysphagia also can be an effect of diffuse cerebrocortical disease. In older patients there may be no other demonstrable neurologic deficits, but there is usually a pattern of "soft signs" of central nervous system disintegration together with decompensation in meeting daily needs. Cineradiologic swallows in such patients may be similar to those in patients who have specific demonstrable neurologic deficits. The overall pattern shows occasional penetration of swallowed material into the pharyngolaryngeal spaces with varying degrees of aspiration.

In pseudobulbar dysphagia, the musculature for swallowing may be somewhat weak and uncoordinated. This condition is distinguished from dysphagia secondary to involvement of the lower motoneuron in that patients retain a swallowing reflex even though it may be difficult to stimulate or initiate voluntarily (Table 5.1). On physical examination, signs such as positive bilateral extensor movements of the great toe (Babinski's sign) are found and are consistent with involvement of the upper motoneurons. There is considerable disinhibition of oral reflexes as evidenced by active rooting, sucking, and biting reflexes that frequently interfere with feeding. Palatal and gag reflexes may be present and may be hyperactive. Speech may be harsh and unintelligible, and language expression and comprehension may be impaired. Because pseudobulbar dysphagia frequently results from bilateral damage to upper motoneurons, patients may lose the cortical controls of swallowing. Loss of learning potential and a reduced ability to make sound judgments may also be found in clinical testing. Disorientation and perceptual deficits may also be present. Part of therapeutic management is directed toward compensating for these deficits (Miller and Groher, 1982).

The loss of intellectual control over swallowing may be superimposed upon uncoordinated performance. Because of the wide variance in the contribution of each of these factors, the clinician must be able to use different combinations of treatment strategies. The challenge is to employ the proper

Table 5.1.   Differences between Pseudobulbar Dysphagia and Paralytic Dysphagia.

Factor	Paralytic Dysphagia	Pseudobulbar Dysphagia
Pathology	Lower motoneuron	Upper motoneuron
Swallow reflex	Absent or very weak	Present, slow, or uncoordinated
Intellect	Intact	May be impaired
Oral strength	Poor	May be normal or uncoordinated
Affect	May be labile	Lability is common
Speech	Flaccid dysarthria	Spastic, hypokinetic, or hyperkinetic dysarthria

combination of intellectual controls in an effort to give the swallow reflex a maximal chance of triggering.

Loss of these intellectual controls translates behaviorally into: (1) forgetting to chew and swallow, usually secondary to reduced environmental awareness and/or distractability; (2) poor judgment characterized by excessive bite sizes or a rapid eating rate, making it most difficult to swallow an overly large bolus; (3) failure to adequately clear the oral cavity before the next bite (the phenomenon of squirreling or pouching of food contents may be related to sensory loss); (4) failure to understand feeding directions secondary to aphasia; (5) different degrees of parietal and frontal lobe pathology that interfere with the patient's perception of the food tray or result in inability to sequence the motor act for feeding; (6) an attempt to eat and talk simultaneously, risking aspiration; (7) generalized failure to appreciate the importance of eating that often is interpreted as lack of motivation, as depression, or as failure to cooperate; and (8) inability to organize and initiate a volitional swallow (Miller and Groher, 1982).

Patients with pseudobulbar dysphagia frequently will have a nasogastric tube already in place when a feeding plan is initiated. As stressed earlier, before beginning the program, it is desirable to have the patient in an optimal state of nutrition and hydration. The decompensating effects of nutritional deficiency and dehydration on bilaterally brain-damaged patients can be marked. Some become so decompensated that once they are fed by nasogastric or intravenous routes their ability to swallow improves dramatically. A team should include a physician and dietitian to monitor progress to give the patient the best chance to succeed when oral feeding trials begin.

The First Feeding Trial

As soon as the patient is medically stable, appropriately alert, and cooperative, the first trial feeding can begin. This should be attempted with the nasogastric tube out. It should not be attempted immediately after a nasogastric feeding, as this would take away the advantage of the hunger drive as an important motivator. The presence of a large (greater than 14 French) tube during oral feeding has four negative effects: (1) it is a mechanical interference in a neurologically impaired system; (2) it partially blocks normal nasal airflow, which makes it more difficult to swallow; (3) its presence in the nasal cavity often forces the patient to mouth-breathe, which dries the oral mucosa and interferes with swallowing; and (4) it can cause food to adhere to it and fall off at an unexpected time, and perhaps be aspirated. The difficulty of swallowing around a large nasogastric tube can be appreciated by trying it.

Some patients with pseudobulbar dysfunction may swallow well enough to protect the airway, but fail to maintain an adequate nutritional state. Fatigue, distractions, and dietary factors may contribute to inadequate intake. Intermittent use of the nasogastric tube in the evening can supplement intake. Clinicians should watch for evidence of irritation of the nasal mucosa that can occur with frequent passage of a feeding tube.

Selection of Foods

As with dysphagia paralytica, the principle of maximal stimulation to trigger the reflex should be applied to patients with pseudobulbar dysphagia. "Easy to chew does not mean easy to swallow" (Larsen, 1976). We recommend using foods that maximally stimulate sensory receptors and are of such consistency that they can be swallowed as a single bolus.

Patients with pseudobulbar dysphagia typically report that liquids are more difficult to swallow than solids. A problem with controlling liquids is a most believable complaint for the patient whose swallowing mechanism lacks the proper timing and reflex elicitation due to neurologic impairment. Liquids that unpredictably spill into the pharynx make them particularly bothersome. Fruit juices are somewhat better because they are flavorful. We have had greater success with liquids if they are first frozen into slush form. The slush consistency provides temperature and texture and helps to form a more predictable and therefore more manageable bolus. Another medium for facilitating intake of liquids is gelatin desserts, particularly when they are prepared with less water than usual (finger Jello), or blenderized to the consistency of whipped cream. Food in these forms does not melt rapidly and is moderately manageable in the mouth and pharynx.

Most of these patients do best with solid foods that are of soft consistency. If possible, it helps to select foods in this category that the patient enjoys. If this information is unavailable from the patient, a family member or friend usually can provide it. Foods that are the most enjoyable serve as motivators and are easier to swallow because of their appeal. The clinician always should be cognizant of making the first few bites significant, and using favorite foods can be of assistance.

Food items that have proved to be effective in eliciting swallowing are medium-soft boiled eggs, cottage cheese, and sliced canned peaches (Larsen, 1976). Bergman (1982) listed foods that are tolerated best in the early stages of treatment: mildly sweet and salty foods; gelatin; poached, boiled, or scrambled eggs; clear soups; broccoli, beets, carrots, peas, and beans; egg and tuna salad; and gravy. She goes on to list foods that are difficult to eat, including such items as hamburger patties, plums, prunes, mashed potatoes, cola-flavored carbonated beverages, all crackers except biscuits, and onions. We recommend that medications should be given in custard, jelly, or blenderized flavored gelatin rather than in an applesauce mixture because of the latter's tendency to fall apart during swallowing. Sticky foods, dry substances, mucus producers, and boluses that fall apart should be avoided.

The patient may tend to use poor judgment by attempting to wash down a solid bolus with liquids. This practice can lead to aspiration if the bolus has either been inadequately masticated or has become lodged in the valleculae. Even mixing liquids with solids in a single bite can confuse the sensory receptors of brain-damaged patients and result in a choking episode.

Intellectual Controls

Selecting the correct diet must be combined with providing the intellectual controls the patient may lack. Therefore, all beginning feedings will require direct assistance aimed at providing the necessary cortical inputs to get a patient swallowing safely.

The first step in providing these controls is to reduce the number of environmental distractions that tend to draw the patient's attention from eating. The first set of distractions is patient-generated. For instance, discomfort due to an improperly positioned arm can serve as enough distraction to focus attention away from eating. If the patient is in pain, prescribed analgesics should be taken well before the meal so that their comforting effect is felt by mealtime. All prosthetic aids should be working and fitting properly, otherwise they are a constant source of distraction. Patients with heavy mucous secretions should have thorough suctioning before meals. Papain, found in most meat tenderizers, can be used on a glycerin swab to thin thick secretions. The oral cavity may need to be cleaned with a fresh swab or toothbrush to stimulate saliva flow and provide needed moisture. In short, the patient should be as comfortable as possible before eating.

The second set of distractions comes from outside sources such as other patients, staff, televisions, and radios. Turning off the television and radio, pulling curtains, and closing doors or facing the patient toward the wall all help the dysphagic individual concentrate on swallowing. The importance of minimizing these distractions in preparation for swallowing should not be overlooked. We have seen patients who complain at initial feedings about discomfort from leg braces, hand splints, condom catheters, or intravenous apparatus. It was impossible to focus their attention on feeding because of these distractions. Clinicians who have made the effort to rehabilitate patients with bilateral brain pathology can attest to the importance of reducing distractions as a prerequisite for learning.

The Feeding Process

After the patient has been properly settled in an upright position, head slightly forward with neck flexed, the feeding process can be initiated (Figure 5.4). (See Chapter 6 for additional detail.) The clinician should avoid long explanations of what is to be expected and accomplished, as these often serve to add confusion to brain-damaged patients, particularly those with language deficits. For the same reason, excessive verbal and gestural cueing by the clinician during feeding should be avoided. In most cases, the patient will know this person is there to assist with feeding and that is sufficient.

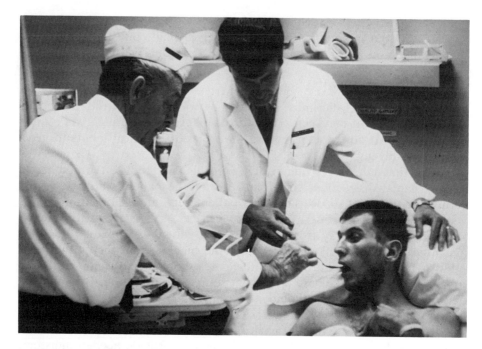

Figure 5.4. Bedridden patient is positioned properly for oral intake with the assistance of a trained volunteer.

The feeding process begins with the patient or feeder loading the utensil with a medium-sized bite (about 15 cc). Bites smaller than this may not create enough pressure to trigger the reflex easily. It often helps to let the patient see and smell the bolus before placing it midway into the oral cavity. This helps to prepare the mechanism for swallowing and is not unlike what happens with normal eating. Immediate assessment of what the patient does with the bolus should be made.

Cognitive cues will have to be provided as necessary. Some patients need verbal or gestural cueing to chew; some need to be told when to swallow; others need to be reminded that food has remained in their mouth and that it must be swallowed before another bite is taken. At this point, it is important to let the patient know when the desired sequence of motor behaviors have been performed (Hargrove, 1980). Constant reinforcement of correct behaviors assists the patient in retaining what has been learned.

The clinician should carefully observe each swallow, paying particular attention to the moment of laryngeal elevation. If the patient prematurely tires or loses interest, there must be no attempt to force feed as it will only frustrate both clinician and patient (Hargrove, 1980). If the patient progresses satisfactorily, the clinician should begin to eliminate specific cues and observe for evidence of compensations in behavior and improved judgment while eating. Some patients will not make these generalizations, and family members or other attendants must be trained to provide the proper input at each meal.

Patients who demonstrate active biting and rooting reflexes that can interfere with placement of utensils often do well if they are allowed to feed themselves. If motor control does not allow this, we recommend a trial with finger foods in measured bites that can be placed in the mouth without utensils or reflex inhibition techniques as described in Chapter 6.

Many patients need an excessive amount of time to complete a meal. Because of the time factor, foods tend to become cold and unappetizing and therefore less stimulating. Patients in this stage of swallowing management benefit from smaller portions given more frequently.

MYASTHENIA GRAVIS

Because myasthenia gravis involves the striated musculature, it may compromise swallowing. Its predilection for the bulbar nuclei and accompanying dysphagia are common.

An estimated 33 percent of patients with myasthenia have significant deglutitory disorders due to fatigue following mastication (Murray, 1962; Silbiger, Pikielney, and Donner, 1967).

Because of this tendency for the musculature to fatigue easily after repeated exercise, patients typically do well at the beginning of a meal, but tire at the end (Merritt, 1967). Mastication and swallowing may be normal and then deteriorate to the point at which there is total loss of the ability to chew and swallow. Continued attempts at feeding past this point can lead to significant aspiration.

Murray (1962) demonstrated by cinefluoroscopy that tongue movements were slow and weak and continued to weaken with additional attempts at swallowing. Holding the bolus on the tongue was particularly troublesome. He studied 23 with disease ranging from mild to severe. Most had barium residual in the oropharynx and valleculae because the tongue failed to arch backward and down into the pharynx. Patients with moderate to severe disease could not clear the valleculae on repeated attempts. There was no evidence of myasthenia affecting the cricopharyngeal sphincter, a finding that Silbiger and colleagues (1967) and Donner and Siegel (1965) supported. Kramer et al. (1957), however, reported on two patients whose cricopharyngeus tired as quickly as their tongue and pharynx. Using cinefluorography, Donner and Siegel (1965) noted the marked fatigability of the tongue and pharyngeal musculature on repeated swallowing attempts. The pharyngeal walls showed prolonged barium coating with pharyngeal recess pooling and loss of tone. Repeated swallowing in some patients produced nasal regurgitation because the pharynx failed to rise adequately to seal the nasopharyngeal port.

The observation that myasthenics have difficulty holding a bolus on the tongue suggests that patients may do better if they are given foods that do not fall apart easily during mastication. Such foods require more lingual effort and hasten fatigue.

Typically, patients with myasthenia are given anticholinesterase-producing drugs that, when administered in the proper doses, greatly facilitate muscle movement. It is important that these medications be coordinated with feeding times so as to facilitate swallowing. If possible, patients should be reminded to limit physical activity before a meal in an effort to maintain sufficient strength to complete it. Such activity can range from strenuous physical therapy to excessive talking. Conservation of energy in the early stages of dysphagia often can be the difference between oral or nasogastric feeding.

AMYOTROPHIC LATERAL SCLEROSIS

Amyotrophic lateral sclerosis (ALS) is a progressive disease of the upper and lower motoneurons of unknown cause and without known treatment. In some cases the deterioration of ALS is confined to muscles supplied by the spinal cord, and dysphagia is not a complication. In a significant number of patients, however, bulbar muscles are also involved and the patient experiences serious difficulties with swallowing.

Clinical findings in the ALS patient with bulbar involvement show a combination of spasticity and flaccidity. In the bulbar muscles specifically, the muscles of mastication (particularly the pterygoids) develop weakness that is experienced as chewing fatigue. The facial muscles (particularly the orbicularis oris) may become weak and drooling is common. The tongue is frequently affected and may look like a "bag of worms" (Blount, Bratton, and Luttrell, 1979) because of muscle fasciculations. As atrophy continues, the tongue weakens and may eventually be paralyzed. Palatal and pharyngeal weakness is common. Speech is hypernasal and may be marked by emission of nasal air. Nasal regurgitation on swallowing is possible, but is not a common finding. The gag reflexes may range from hyperactive in one patient to absent in another. An intact gag can disappear during the course of the disease. The muscles that elevate the larynx may develop weakness and the cricopharyngeus may fail to relax during swallowing. Some patients complain of cramping in various muscle groups, occasionally in the suprahyoid muscles. Weakness of vocal folds in our experience usually causes incomplete abduction that restricts breathing. Vocal fold adduction is incomplete and the folds appear bowed as they meet. Respiratory insufficiency and weakness of abdominal muscles lead to a poor protective cough. Sensation is not affected and most patients retain good cognitive function.

Since the dysphagia of ALS generally is progressive and the symptoms are highly variable, establishing a baseline of function and following the patient throughout the course of the disease is recommended. The baseline data should include a thorough clinical dysphagia examination (see Chapter 4). Some centers advocate following patients with a series of cineradiographic studies (Bosma and Brodie, 1969).

Management of dysphagia should begin early in the course of the disease. Patients will need to be instructed to eat in an upright posture with the neck flexed (DeLisa et al., 1979). Foods that cause problems should be noted so that the consistency of the diet can be controlled. As expected, fluids are more easily aspirated than solids. Most blenderized foods act like liquid and fall apart in the mouth and pharynx. Therefore soft foods such as macaroni casseroles and custard work well. As with other dysphagic patients, sticky food and substances that combine with saliva to cause thick mucus should be minimized in the diet.

As the disease progresses, the management of nutrition by oral feeding may become unsafe. Aspiration pneumonitis is a major cause of death in ALS. It is the dysphagia specialist's role to recommend procedures that may improve swallowing or alternative methods of providing nutrition. Lebo, Sang, and Norris (1976) reported that 64 percent of their patients had improved swallowing following cricopharyngeal myotomy. Although the benefits from this procedure may only be temporary, the quality of the patients' lives may be enhanced.

Timing is very important when recommending alternatives to swallowing. Most patients desire to maintain oral intake of food and liquid for as long as possible; however, those who quit eating and drinking for even short periods of time may become too weak to withstand surgical intervention. Others have severely compromised respiratory systems predisposing them to surgical complications. When the gag reflex permits, intermittent oral placement of a feeding tube for nutritional support is the best alternative to swallowing. If this is not well tolerated, cervical esophagostomy has proved to be successful.

Clinicians who offer symptomatic management for patients with progressive motoneuron disease should realize that the clinical course is highly variable and, so far, unpredictable. Although the symptoms cannot be arrested or prevented, the support offered by the dysphagia specialist may go far in improving the quality of the patient's remaining life.

HUNTINGTON'S CHOREA

Some of the feeding problems of patients with Huntington's chorea are unique to this disease, while others are typical of patients with pseudobulbar dysphagia. The characteristic choreatic movements of Huntington's disease eventually severely compromise feeding and swallowing. At the time of diagnosis, feeding and swallowing disorders are infrequent. As the disease progresses, however, and the involuntary movements become more frequent and uncontrollable, dysphagia emerges as a significant problem. The constant movements cause a significant number of calories to be burned, and patients frequently have appetites that are difficult to satisfy; their focus on food and eating becomes paramount. Difficulty with oral intake conflicts with their unsatisfied hunger and creates a significant feeding management problem. For some patients, their frustrations are compounded by documented changes in mental status that interfere with the ability to learn compensatory feeding and swallowing strategies.

Typically, patients first lose the ability to manipulate utensils for self-feeding and require direct assistance in food transport. Once food and liquids are placed in the mouth they usually are managed without great difficulty. At this stage, some patients prefer to remain independent in feeding and therefore exercise the option of increasing the number of food items that can be consumed without utensils such as sandwiches, fruits, and selected vegetables.

As the choreatic movements intensify, there is marked involvement in the coordination of swallowing. In addition, unpredictable, sudden gulps of air during the inspiratory cycle open the glottis at irregular intervals, compromising protection of the airway. The head may suddenly be thrust back, exposing the airway. Because of the characteristic writhing tongue, lateralization and posterior transportation of food toward the pharynx are difficult. Forming the posterior bolus needed to trigger a swallowing reflex becomes an obstacle in completing a normal swallow (Kilman, 1977). Foods and liquids reach the oropharynx with unpredictable speed. We can postulate that such irregular control may create abnormal timing sequences that invite laryngeal penetration and aspiration.

Over a five-year period, Groher had the opportunity to follow six patients with advanced Huntington's disease and swallowing complaints. All patients were hospitalized, nonambulatory, and could not meet most of their daily needs, including self-feeding. Four of the six had accompanying changes in mental status such as poor judgment, uncontrollable outbursts of temper, and disorientation. Their mean age was 47.6 years. All patients had had the disease for 12 years or more.

The patients were evaluated for their dysphagia complaints. At the time of the evaluation, all were receiving their nutrition orally; however, fluoroscopic evidence of increased laryngeal penetration suggested they should receive a complete dysphagia work-up. None had demonstrable aspiration pneumonia, although the nurses reported considerable choking, sputtering, and prolonged coughing at mealtimes. All six were eating pureed foods and not one was satisfied with this diet. The swallowing evaluation consistently revealed the following: (1) the nursing assistant who was feeding the patient had great difficulty placing the food in the patient's mouth due to marked choreatic movements of the head and trunk; (2) once the food was placed, the tongue often pushed the bolus anteriorly out of the mouth; (3) oral mastication was labored and the time between oral placement and a swallow reflex was not consistent, frequently being either too fast or delayed;

(4) laryngeal elevation during swallowing was normal; (5) solids were managed better than liquids; (6) all had protective coughs; (7) all swallowed a soft mechanical diet without difficulty; and (8) all swallowed more efficiently when the environment was free of distraction (measured by less coughing and shorter total mealtime).

The evaluation revealed that the most crucial phase of swallowing management in patients with Huntington's disease took place in the preparatory stages of swallowing. For instance, two of six patients could not maintain a proper position for effective swallowing. This was managed as well as possible by providing head and trunk restraints during meals. Such restraints, of course, did not reduce the choreatic movements, but did help patients to maintain upright posture. Spoon feeding was accomplished best when the feeder did not try to introduce the spoon at his or her will, but rather held the spoon in front of the patients waiting for them to take the food from it. Allowing the patient to take the food voluntarily resulted in fewer incidences of the tongue pushing the bolus out of the oral cavity. Finally, all patients were more motivated to eat because they received a diet that was more pleasing to their senses and equally as easy to swallow.

PARKINSON'S DISEASE

Another variant of pseudobulbar symptomatology is seen in patients with Parkinson's disease. The clinical features of tremor and rigidity may precipitate swallowing dysfunction. Like those with Huntington's chorea, patients with Parkinson's disease become progressively handicapped, and it is not until the final stages of the disease, when rigidity is the prominent feature, that dysphagia becomes a significant management problem (Lieberman et al., 1980).

A review of the literature seems to suggest a wide variability as to the prevalence and type of swallowing disorder that Parkinson's disease precipitates. Undoubtedly, the discrepancies exist due to subject selection (lack of clarity of disease stages) and the positioning of the patient during radiographic studies. Whether or not abnormal cineradiographic studies correlate with the severity of the disease or with the significance of the dysphagia still remains a primary question. That this question remains unanswered challenges the clinician to design individualized treatment plans rather than generalize to all patients with Parkinson's disease.

Lieberman and associates (1980) contended that some degree of dysphagia may be present in 50 percent of cases, but is rarely so severe as to require gastrostomy. Eadie and Tyrer (1965) reported a similar figure, and our clinical experience suggests that most patients are able to take nutrition orally, even in the end stages of disease. Eadie and Tyrer (1965) found no correlation between severity of disease and severity of dysphagia. Their findings are supported by Lieberman and his colleagues (1980) who studied two cases with end-stage disease; one had adequate voice and tongue mobility but aspirated, and one had poor voice and tongue movement but did not aspirate.

The results of cineradiography are conflicting. Silbiger and associates (1967) found swallowing abnormalities in all 11 patients studied. Abnormalities were described as poor bolus formation, misdirected swallow, abnormal pharyngeal motility, pharyngeal stasis, and abnormal cricopharyngeal function. Eadie and Tyrer (1965) examined 107 patients and found that dysphagia existed secondary to faulty control of the pharyngeal constrictors. Palmer (1974) reported that the dysphagia associated with Parkinson's disease usually was due to hypopharyngeal dysfunction, and recommended relief with posterior cricopharyngeal sphincterotomy. Calne and associates (1970) studied 20 patients and found no pharyngeal pathology. They attributed the differences between their studies and Silbiger's to the fact that the latter studied patients in the prone position rather than sitting upright. Calne et al. (1970) concluded that parkinsonian dysphagia was more related to oral and/or esophageal disorders, as they had noted lingual hesitancy and piecemeal deglutition in the oral stages. Logemann et al. (1977) presented cineradiographic evidence showing that regardless of the stage of disease, patients have slowed oral and esophageal transit times.

We can conclude from these investigations that swallowing disorders in parkinsonism may be present in varying degrees and combinations in the oropharyngeal complex, and that the severity of the movement disorder probably does not correlate with the severity of the dysphagia. In addition, it has not been established whether or not abnormal cineradiographic studies give an accurate prognostication for clinical aspiration. They can, however, suggest appropriate treatment strategies.

Calne and associates (1970) found fluoroscopic evidence in these patients of lingual hesitancy causing poor bolus formation; this is also evident clinically. Patients frequently take excessive time to masticate and manipulate the bolus in the oral cavity before swallowing. Tongue and mandibular excursions are limited and formation of a posterior bolus is difficult. Once a swallow reflex is triggered, the larynx rises normally. It is reasonable to assume that the difficulty experienced in oral bolus formation and anteroposterior mobility creates timing mismatches between the oral and pharyngeal phases not unlike those seen in patients with mechanical swallowing disorders secondary to tongue lesions (Logemann and Bytell, 1979).

Because of the excessive time taken for oral mastication, it is more advantageous for patients to eat smaller portions more frequently, especially if feeding times are restricted. Changing the portions and increasing the length of mealtimes have two distinct psychologic advantages. First, patients feel they do not need to finish a large portion in a short time and therefore enjoy their meals more. Second, they are aware they will not be left hungry if they do not finish one large meal in a fixed time segment. These facilitators are important motivators for swallowing.

In our experience, patients with Parkinson's disease generally do well with regular diets. In the end stages of disease, they find it easier to eat soft foods that require less effort to masticate. Teaching a more posterior spoon placement often is helpful in reducing oral transit times, but patients must avoid bypassing sensory receptors that help trigger the swallow reflex.

The timing of dopaminergic medications should coincide with mealtimes so that their effect can facilitate oral and pharyngeal movements. Such an effect will vary from patient to patient depending on drug dosage and individual metabolic rates. Lieberman and associates (1980) pointed out that it is important to have patients swallow their medications because parenteral anticholinergics are not as effective as levodopa taken orally. The usefulness of levodopa in alleviating dysphagic symptoms remains controversial, however. Some patients have benefited, while others have not (Cotzias, Papavalilion, and Gellene, 1969; Calne et al., 1970; Lieberman et al., 1980).

SUMMARY

This chapter contains some general treatment guidelines for patients who suffer from dysphagia secondary to neurologic impairments. Specific treatment and pretreatment considerations for this group are covered in the following chapter.

The clinician must remain cognizant of the fact that signs and symptoms of neurologic pathology may change over time. In addition, well described disease entities and processes affect patients in differing ways. Therefore, we should not lose sight of the fact that dysphagia management with this group of patients is predicated on individualized plans.

REFERENCES

Bergman K. Dysphagia in the adult patient. Conference on rehabilitation of dysphagia in adults. Detroit, Michigan, July 29 and 30, 1982.

Blount M, Bratton C, Luttrell N. Management of the patient with amyotrophic lateral sclerosis. Nurs Clin North Am 1979;14:157–71.

Bonanno PC. Swallowing dysfunction after tracheostomy. Ann Surg 1971;174:29–33.

Bosma JF, Brodie DR. Disabilities of the pharynx in ALS as demonstrated by cineradiography. Radiology 1969;92:97–103.

Calne DB, Shaw DG, Spiers ASD, Stern GM. Swallowing in parkinsonism. Br J Radiol 1970;43:456–57.

Cotzias GC, Papavalilion PS, Gellene R. Modification of parkinsonism—chronic treatment with L-dopa. N Engl J Med 1969;280:337–45.

DeLisa JA, Mikulic MA, Miller RM, Melnick RR. Amyotrophic lateral sclerosis: comprehensive management. Am Fam Physician 1979;19:137–42.

Donner MW, Siegel CI. The evaluation of pharyngeal neuromuscular disorders by cinefluorography. Am J Roentgenol 1965;94:299–307.

Eadie MJ, Tyrer JH. Alimentary disorders in parkinsonism. Aust Ann Med 1965;14:13–22.

English GM, Morfit HM, Ratzer ER. Cervical esophagostomy in head and neck cancer. Arch Otolaryngol 1970;92:335–39.

Hargrove R. Feeding the severely involved patient. J Neurosurg Nurs 1980;12:102–7.

Kilman WJ. Diseases of the pharynx and larynx. Curr Probl Diagn Radiol 1977;7:1–43.

Kramer P, Atkinson M, Wyman SM, Ingelfinger FJ. The dynamics of swallowing. II. Neuromuscular dysphagia of the pharynx. J Clin Invest 1957;36:589–95.

Larsen GL. Rehabilitating dysphagia: mechanica, paralytica, pseudobulbar. J Neurosurg Nurs 1976;8:14–17.

Lebo CP, Sang UK, Norris FH. Cricopharyngeal myotomy in amyotrophic lateral sclerosis. Laryngoscope 1976;86:862–68.

Lieberman AM, Horowitz L, Redmond P, Pachter L, Lieberman I, Leibowitz M. Dysphagia in Parkinson's disease. Am J Gastroenterol 1980;74:157–60.

Lindeman RC. Diverting the paralyzed larynx: a reversible procedure for intractable aspiration. Laryngoscope 1975;85:157–80.

Logemann JA, Boshes B, Blonsky RE, Fisher HE. Speech and swallowing evaluation in the differential diagnosis of neurologic disease. Neurologica-Neurocirugia-Psiquiatria 1977;18:71–8.

Logemann JA, Bytell DE. Swallowing disorders in three types of head and neck surgical patients. Cancer 1979;44:1095–1105.

Merritt HH. A textbook of neurology. Philadelphia: Lea & Febiger, 1967.

Miller RM, Groher ME. The evaluation and management of neuromuscular and mechanical swallowing disorders. Dysarthria, Dysphonia, Dysphagia 1982;1:50–70.

Montgomery WW. Surgery to prevent aspiration. Arch Otolaryngol 1975;101:679–82.

Murray JP. Deglutition in myasthenia gravis. Br J Radiol 1962;35:43–52.

Palmer ED. Dysphagia in parkinsonism. JAMA 1974;229:1349.

Silbiger ML, Pikielney R, Donner MW. Neuromuscular disorders affecting the pharynx: cineradiographic analysis. Invest Radiol 1967;2:442–48.

Smith AC, Spanling JM, Ardran G, Livingstone G. Laryngectomy in the management of severe dysphagia in nonmalignant conditions. Lancet 1965;2:1094–96.

CHAPTER 6

Management of Neurologic Disorders—The First Feeding Session

Ina Elfant Asher

Upon completing a dysphagia evaluation of a patient with a neurologic disorder, several determinations can be made: possible risk of aspiration, whether or not the patient is alert enough for the initiation of prefeeding or swallowing training, and areas of oral and facial impairment that might interfere with swallowing functions. Although a preliminary estimation of prognosis can be made based on the evaluation, only implementation of a course of treatment will determine the patient's ultimate potential for feeding success. The goal may range from independent consumption of a full oral diet to limited oral feeding with nonoral supplements. Sometimes a course of treatment may indicate that the patient is not a good candidate for oral feeding, in which case more appropriate recommendations can be made.

This chapter offers a regimen for beginning a swallowing training program. General prefeeding management of the neurogenic dysphagia patient is discussed, followed by a description of the initial feeding session. Additional considerations and adaptations of the program that are specific to the neurologic population are included. Finally, for those patients who require additional devices or equipment to enable them to feed themselves more independently, special aids are described.

PREFEEDING MANAGEMENT

Alertness

Alertness and cooperation are the first requirements of a patient embarking on a dysphagia treatment program. Lethargy during training and inattention during swallowing increase the risk of aspiration. For this reason, general stimulation techniques can be used to improve the patient's mental status. The room should be well-lit and the patient assisted to a proper upright sitting position (as described later). A favorable time of day should be chosen for sessions depending on individual habits and hospital routine. For example, it is wise to avoid scheduling sessions following physical therapy, lengthy test procedures (x-rays, scans), or a tube feeding, when the patient is not hungry.

The dysphagia therapist should attempt, as should all hospital personnel involved in the patient's care, to orient the patient and explain the purpose of treatment. If confusion or disorientation persists, the patient should be reminded of the surroundings and the status of the present feeding problem.

Multisensory stimulation can be used to improve alertness, for example, visual and auditory stimulation from the environment. Rhythmic music, variations in the therapist's voice and manner, and a lighted, colorful room will have a stimulating effect on the patient. Compare this to a dull, drab room with lowered voices and slow repetitive music that can promote relaxation and sleep. Stimulation must be planned and orderly, however. A noisy, cluttered, and bustling area with many interruptions and constantly changing activity can be overstimulating and confusing, or have a disorganizing effect on the treatment session (Ayres, 1973; Trombly and Scott, 1977).

Sensory Impairment

When oral or facial sensation is impaired, the patient must be made aware of the type and extent of impairment. This may be done cognitively, that is, relying on the patient's understanding and ability to adapt to the new situation, or through specific techniques of stimulation or inhibition. On the conscious level, safety precautions can be emphasized to prevent the injury of sensitive mucous membranes from hot foods, biting, or other injury.

Food should be placed initially in the most sensitive area of the mouth for protection as well as maximum stimulation to taste, temperature, and texture. If food is frequently retained in the sensory-impaired side of the mouth or if unchecked drooling is noted, inattention to the involved side may be a factor. In this case, use of a mirror, verbal cues by the trainer, and frequent checks inside the mouth for food squirreled away are necessary. Although directing food to the unimpaired side of the mouth is one method of compensating, a patient may not change habits so easily. In fact, the hemiplegic may tend to chew on the involved side more frequently. It is desirable for the patient to learn to perform these checks in order to handle food on both sides of the mouth.

Sometimes the skin of a brain-damaged adult becomes hypersensitive to various types of facial stimulation. This can be observed by aversive reactions (noted in facial expression or shying away) to such stimuli as light, moving touch or sustained touch. The muscles underlying the hypersensitive skin may also be affected. If hypersensitivity occurs, Farber (1982) recommends applying maintained pressure to the perioral area (such as firm placement of the finger horizontally across the maxilla between the nose and upper lip), pressure to the cheeks and temples if necessary, and once the patient is calmed, maintained pressure to dorsum of the tongue with a rubber seizure stick in the midline about one-third of the way back on the tongue. A device is easily made by occupational therapists by molding lip-shaped thermoplastic splinting material around a padded tongue blade or a rubber seizure stick (Figure 6.1).

Hygiene

The teeth and gums of the dysphagic patient should be well cared for and cleansed. Dried secretions often accumulate on the tongue and palate, reducing oral sensitivity and promoting growth of bacteria in the mouth. Lemon-glycerine swabs are often used to refresh and cleanse the mouth. They are also useful as a sensory stimulant as they are cold, wet, and tart in flavor. If an adverse reaction to the strong flavor is noticed, the swab may be rinsed to dilute the taste. If the secretions are quite thick or hardened in the oral cavity, they should be gently but regularly removed with a damp washcloth.

The patient who wears dentures should continue to do so, and the

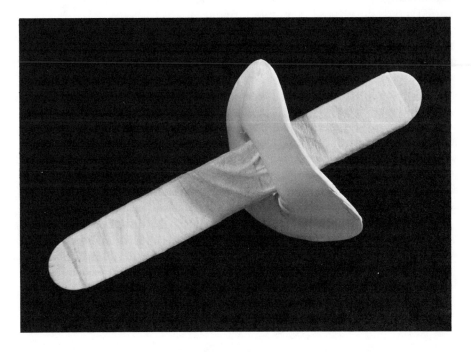

Figure 6.1. Modified seizure stick can be used to apply pressure to the tongue dorsum to inhibit hypersensitivity.

dentures should be regularly cleansed. Illness should not alter the fit of the dentures. Many denture wearers, however, use their oral muscles to hold poorly fitted dentures in place. If the oral musculature is weak, the dentures may appear to be looser.

Muscle Tone

Some patients with upper motoneuron disease may display spasticity or abnormalities of muscle tone that are persistent or severe enough to interfere with normal swallowing. To illustrate this influence, one need only hunch one shoulder into a shrug as hard as possible and then try to swallow. Changes in tone may indicate a dominating influence of primitive postural reflexes that can reappear in the brain-damaged adult. For example, the asymmetric tonic neck reflex will cause a change in muscle tone in the limbs when the head is turned to one side. The limbs on the side toward which the head is facing show an increase in extensor tone and the jaw may deviate in that direction (Mueller, 1975). In the tonic labyrinthine reflex, a supine position in bed can increase extensor tone in the body (Fiorentino, 1974). Thus in addition to increased muscle tension in the neck and trunk that can interfere with ease of swallowing, an increase in neck extension can invite aspiration by increasing oral access to the airway. Proper positioning for feeding sessions can largely reduce these primitive influences.

In some patients with upper motoneuron lesions, optimal positioning is difficult, and treatment should be coordinated with or preceded by therapy with a trained occupational or physical therapist to normalize muscle tone. If tone is found to be excessive, causing muscle tension, resistance to free movement, and stiffness of posture, techniques of muscle inhibition can be used to relax the patient. This may include slow and repetitive stroking of body parts, rocking, and maintaining firm pressures on specific muscle and skin areas. Once desired relaxation is achieved, facilitatory techniques such as joint compression, quick muscle stretch, light touch over skin or muscle areas, high-frequency vibration or manual tapping over the muscle fibers, and resistance to movement may be selectively applied. Facilitation techniques can improve muscle tone, strengthen desired motions, and redistribute the balance of muscle power for posture when applied to reciprocal muscle groups (Trombly and Scott, 1977). Such methods should only be attempted by personnel trained in their use due to the complexity of the techniques and their consequences to entire body function and movement. Used properly, they can prepare a patient for normal oral function.

Weakness

Oral and facial weakness can impair the function of the swallowing mechanism itself as well as the accessory structures (lips, buccal or cheek, tongue, jaw) that form and manipulate the bolus for chewing and swallowing. For example, if the muscles of lip closure, the orbicularis oris superior and inferior, are weak, food and liquid will leak out since the lips will not maintain a tightly closed position. Treatment must include strengthening of these structures (Silverman and Elfant, 1979). Lip and facial exercises are summarized as follows:

1. Broad smiling with lips closed and open
2. Tight frowning
3. Alternate lip pursing and retraction
4. Practice producing words and sounds: u, m, b, p, w
5. Resistive sucking on a pinched straw
6. Blowing up cheeks with mouth tightly closed to prevent escaping air
7. Blowing exercises: match, cotton ball, candle, straw, whistle
8. Hard sucking on frozen popsicle
9. Pursing lips around a button tied on a string, gradually reducing button size

The exercises can be done in front of a mirror to promote awareness of facial symmetry, especially in the event of sensory loss. To strengthen lip closure further, the therapist can apply manual vibration to the orbicularis oris muscles followed by quick stretch in the direction away from contraction (Farber, 1982). Huffman (1978) used electromyographic feedback on the orbicularis oris muscles to retrain lip movements. Coordinating biofeedback with exercises in front of a mirror resulted in greater and faster gains in movement.

If the patient has difficulty following directions for different positions, words should be used that indicate a familiar action, such as "blow" or "kiss" instead of "purse your lips." This appeals to subcortical performance to elicit a desired movement, and a mirror may prove to be a hindrance.

Jaw Control

Jaw stability must be maintained for normal sucking and chewing to take place. If the chin juts out in jaw protraction, the therapist can pull out quickly on the jaw and then hold it out to stimulate the muscles of retraction. If the problem is overretraction, the therapist pushes in on the chin quickly and has the patient hold it in with resistance to stimulate the opposite motion for protraction (Farber, 1982).

To prepare the patient for chewing and to strengthen jaw motions prior to the introduction of food, a gauze-wrapped tongue depressor may be used. It is most stimulating if dampened with flavoring, such as cranberry juice (tart flavor stimulates salivation and sucking). For the patient without teeth or dentures in place, dried fruit or gumdrops suspended on a string are effective for gumming. These should be removed at any sign of particles breaking off.

Tongue Movements

To strengthen tongue movements, active and resistive exercises should be performed for the motions of tongue retraction, protraction, lateralization, elevation, and depression. General exercises include:

1. Pronounce "la la la," "ta ta ta," d, n, z, s.
2. Push against a tongue depressor in varying directions both inside and outside the mouth.
3. Lick or push the tongue tip against a lollipop.
4. Count the teeth with the tongue.
5. Push the tongue against the inner wall of the cheeks as hard as possible.
6. Push the tongue tip against the roof of the mouth and against the lower teeth.
7. Lick a sticky substance from the roof of the mouth.
8. Protrude the tongue and lick off small amounts of jelly placed on the lips.

Speech

When weakness in the oral structures exists, dysarthria often accompanies dysphagia. If treatment is coordinated with the speech pathologist, both problems can be addressed. The therapist should be aware, however, that some articulation skills may not be equivalents but rather complements to eating and swallowing skills, as in movements of the mandible during chewing versus speaking (Bosma, 1970). Therefore strengthening one may not have the same effect on the other.

Oral Reflexes

The oral reflexes of adults can be divided into two categories: those that are normal (e.g., cough, gag) and those that are abnormal (e.g., rooting, bite, tongue thrust). If the gag reflex is not elicited in testing or is found to be weak, facilitation techniques should be attempted to induce or strengthen these important protective responses prior to feeding. In addition, the swallowing reflex should be facilitated or practiced if it is not readily performed either spontaneously or to command. Inhibitory techniques may be used to inhibit abnormal reflexes that interfere with attempts at feeding.

Normal Reflexes

To stimulate the gag reflex or strengthen it (i.e., elicit a stronger and more consistent response to testing), the palatoglossal and palatopharyngeal arches, uvula, soft palate, and posterior tongue are lightly stroked with a tongue depressor or rubber seizure stick (Silverman and Elfant, 1979). This is repeated several times or until a gag is elicited, and can be repeated several times daily as it is quick and easy to do. Pressure or jabbing motions lateral to this area are to be avoided because of the close proximity of the carotid vessels.

Swallowing stimulation techniques are used when the patient is not consistently swallowing during testing or able voluntarily to swallow to command. Since dry swallows (swallowing without food or liquid in the mouth) are difficult to execute, stimulation techniques should be carried out using a lollipop, ice pop, or several drops of cold water from an eye dropper. A rinse with a lemon-glycerine swab to stimulate salivation is a good alternative.

To induce swallowing, several maneuvers may be tried (Silverman and Elfant, 1979). These include:

1. Application of an ice cube for two or three seconds to the sternal notch during the attempted swallow (wrap the ice to prevent dripping).
2. Gentle upward stroking under the chin with the therapist's fingers.
3. Manual vibration of the laryngopharyngeal musculature, starting under the chin and vibrating down either side of the larynx to the notch.
4. Actively tilting the head forward as the patient prepares to swallow.
5. Application of stretch pressure to pharyngeal constrictor muscles by manual traction applied (from behind) with the heels of the hands to the base of the skull in a forward and upward direction.

When the act of swallowing can be consistently elicited either to command or to stimulation, feeding may be attempted. The ability to swallow is, after all, the primary indication of readiness to eat. Although other functions such as the gag reflex, good oral sensation, and adequate tongue mobility are desirable, it is possible to eat safely without them. Precautions should always be taken to compensate for remaining dysfunction, and supplementary treatment should continue with feeding training.

Abnormal Reflexes

The abnormal oral reflexes should be inhibited if possible, as they can interfere with attempts to eat. We may differentiate between the reflexes that are abnormal at any age, such as tongue thrust and bite reflex, and those that are normal in infants but should not be exhibited after the first few months of life, such as rooting and mouth opening. Although reflexes in the latter category may interfere less with swallowing training, it is desirable to achieve normal control in all aspects of eating. Some primitive or infantile reflexes may actually aid the brain-damaged adult in eating. In the suck-swallow reflex, swallowing is triggered reflexively by sucking. Again, the goal is to achieve normal eating patterns, free of primitive reflex control.

One method for reducing interference of abnormal oral reflexes is to avoid eliciting them (Silverman and Elfant, 1979). If a bite reflex exists, stimulation of the molar or gum surfaces or the masseter muscles should be avoided. If the patient clamps the teeth onto the spoon, one should not pull or pry the mouth open, but wait for spontaneous opening to occur. Pressure to the temporomandibular joint thrusting the jaw forward can also induce mouth opening. To avoid eliciting the rooting reflex, one must not touch the cheek or corners of the mouth. The mouth-opening reflex is triggered by the visual appearance of an approaching spoon or object (not always food) and is therefore difficult to avoid. For this reason, the therapist can try to direct mouth opening verbally in advance of presenting the food and thus encourage the response at a cortical level ("Would you like lime Jello? Open your mouth, please, and I will give you some"). These reflexes will often diminish spontaneously.

There are some techniques that are used to actually inhibit reflexes (Farber, 1982). Proper positioning is the foremost method. As discussed, it helps to reduce the effect of abnormal postural tone and brainstem reflexes. With proper posturing, the bite reflex may be less active; it may be further inhibited by maintained pressure on the tongue with a rubber seizure stick.

The gag reflex can become hyperactive in the brain-damaged adult. Thus, excessive gagging may result from the stimulation provided by food. To inhibit the reflex, constant pressure is applied with a rubber seizure stick to the dorsum of the tongue, midline about one-third of the way back. The pressure should be maintained for three to five seconds and repeated several times to reduce hypersensitivity. Walking back firmly and slowly on the tongue several times with a tongue depressor until just before the reflex is elicited may also reduce hyperactivity. Techniques to reduce facial hyper-sensitivity described earlier frequently help to normalize oral hypersensitivity and the overreactive gag reflex.

The tongue thrust may be counteracted by facilitating the tongue's opposite motion, retracting or drawing back (Silverman and Elfant, 1979; Farber, 1982). To stimulate tongue retraction, pressure can be applied under the chin to the tongue retraction muscles. Manual vibration may be done with the forefinger or a rubber seizure stick on either side of the frenulum under the tongue. Retraction can be strengthened by resistive sucking, such as picking up bits of paper with the end of a straw.

Sucking may be a primitive reflex if the patient is unable to begin or stop sucking at will, but is dependent upon presentation or removal of the stimulus (straw, lollipop, ice pop) to do so, or if it cannot be isolated from a suck-swallow sequence. Although it is desirable to bring sucking to a level of cortical control, the sucking reflex can be used in early stages of treatment to elicit a reflexive swallow when a voluntary swallow is absent. Pressure on the tip of the tongue has been suggested to elicit automatic sucking and reduce drooling (Trombly and Scott, 1977). Farber (1982) recommended a simple device to promote swallowing that can be constructed from a plastic squeeze bottle, fish tank hose, and Aquaplast (Figure 6.2). The mouthpiece provides maintained pressure over the orbicularis oris to promote sucking while liquid is drawn into the patient's mouth by the vacuum created by the lip seal. The fish tank tube must be bonded to the mouthpiece with a heat gun and its opposite end cut on an angle and inserted snugly into the bottle. For best results, the mouthpiece is molded to the individual patient, indenting it between the lips slightly to make a shelf.

FEEDING TRAINING

As mentioned previously, alertness and the ability to swallow are the critical requirements for eating. If these qualifications are met during the initial

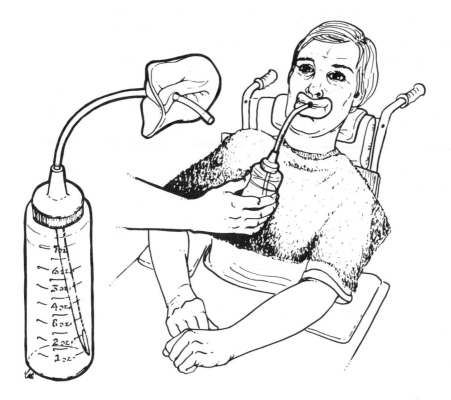

Figure 6.2. A plastic squeeze bottle, fish tank hose, and Aquaplast can be used to promote swallowing behavior. Reprinted by permission of the publisher, from Farber, *Neurorehabilitation: multisensory approach.* Philadelphia: WB Saunders, 1982.

evaluation, a feeding trial may follow. If one or both abilities are not present, oral feedings may be delayed for any length of time while the prefeeding regimen can begin. If tube feedings have been instituted, they should not interfere with the initiation of oral feedings unless large-diameter rigid nasogastric tubes are in place. If this is the case, the patient may experience some discomfort in addition to possible inhibition of the gag reflex. It is preferable to begin training after removal of this type of feeding tube.

Early Precautions

Feeding training requires the candidate to be awake, alert, and cooperative. Every effort must be made to inform the patient verbally or through gestures that the purpose of training is to eat without choking. If language impairment is severe, the patient may not be able to follow instructions or indicate needs or discomforts. In such a case, the feeding session should be structured in a way that simulates familiar eating routines, food preferences, and personal habits. This information can be obtained from the family. In addition, the patient's tolerance to food and symptoms of distress must be watched carefully. Signs of aspiration include: rapid heart rate, sudden change of color (gray), gasping, coughing, hoarse or breathy voice quality, and bubbling or gurgling sounds in the chest (audible or heard with a stethoscope) (Silverman and Elfant, 1979). It is useful to practice auscultation with a stethoscope to become familiar with normal and congested breath sounds. If the patient is congested, dairy products should be avoided as they tend to thicken secretions, while oily substances such as beef broth thin secretions. If aspiration is suspected, the attending physician should be alerted.

If the patient has a tracheostoma tube in place, a methylene blue test (see Chapter 4) should be administered prior to the first feeding session. After drinking a few sips of water dyed with methylene blue, the trachea is suctioned to determine whether aspiration of the stained water has occurred. If it has, oral feeding should not be initiated. The same test can be conducted using methylene blue-stained ice. When the tracheostoma tube has an inflatable cuff, it should be deflated before either test.

For the first feeding session, precautions should be taken against aspiration. Deep suction apparatus and personnel trained in using it should be available. Any incident of acute aspiration should be reported promptly to the appropriate staff. The feeding should be halted and the patient reassured. As this can be a frightening experience, it may cause increased anxiety to both patient and staff at future feeding sessions.

Environment

Early feeding sessions should be conducted in a private setting free of distractions. If possible, the patient should sit upright in a chair, facing the dysphagia therapist. This promotes a more symmetric posture (described in the section on positioning). If the patient is easily distracted, conducting the session in a private room or drawing the curtains to minimize outside stimulation may be necessary. Conversation should be minimal and instructions concise. Even when the patient concentrates well on the task at hand, the feeding session should not be a time for social conversation. The setting should be structured to facilitate good swallowing behavior and careful eating habits.

Positioning

Proper positioning of the patient is essential to promote normal swallowing. The patient should sit upright with legs slightly apart and the hips, knees, and ankles in at least 90 degrees of flexion. The head should be slightly forward (chin tucked) to avoid neck extension. This position helps maintain good alignment with the alimentary tract. If the head is tilted back, alignment is made with the airway, which invites aspiration.

If the patient must remain in bed, a pillow can be placed under the knees; hip and knee flexion helps to counteract the same extensor tone that acts on the neck. The position of forward flexion in bed can be maintained by placing pillows behind the patient's back to support the trunk. Pressure should never be exerted to the back of the head to maintain ventroflexion, as this can elicit the tonic labyrinthine reflex and facilitate a reflex extension of the neck (Farber, 1982). Ensuring a midline position of the head will help to eliminate the influence of another common primitive reflex, the asymmetric tonic neck reflex. The patient should be assisted to maintain as symmetric a posture as possible.

Food Selection and Administration

Although water is highly facilitatory to swallowing, it is poorly controlled by patients with neurogenic dysphagia and is likely to promote choking. In choosing food items for these individuals, texture, taste, temperature, and odor should be considered. The item should be appealing (observe the patient's facial expression for a reaction) and the temperature stimulating (not tepid). My experience suggests that the consistency of the initial food selections should be thick, as the bulk is more easily maneuvered, more readily felt, and more easily controlled. Crumbly textures should be avoided initially so that small bits will not pose a risk for aspiration. Ideal trial foods are gelatin desserts, custard, or pudding.

Test swallows can be made using small amounts of chipped or crushed ice or an ice popsicle. Banana- or vanilla-flavored pops stimulate sucking (Farber, 1982) and put water in a more controllable form as it slowly melts.

In addition, cold temperature is very stimulating to the oral sense receptors. The ice should be offered to the patient in small amounts on a small metal spoon. If the patient chokes on the ice, it may be useful to try swallows using a lollipop (moistened with cold water if the mouth is dry). The sweet lollipop placed in the mouth for sucking will stimulate salivation and taste receptors for swallowing, and is less likely to cause aspiration. If excessive choking followed by aspiration does occur with both items, the patient should not attempt other foods.

If the test swallows are performed comfortably and consistently, trial foods may be administered. A small amount of the gelatin, custard, or pudding is placed on the tip of a small spoon and offered to the patient to see and smell. As the patient opens the mouth, the therapist places the spoon firmly down on the center of the tongue and allows the patient to remove the food with the lips. The pressure of the spoon on the tongue helps to elicit mouth closure and removal of food (Mueller, 1975). Sometimes this effect takes a moment, and the therapist should maintain firm spoon position on the tongue. Spoon placement also helps to keep the head in a lowered midline position. The therapist must always present the food from a low height (never above mouth level) to prevent the patient from raising the head and extending the neck.

Once the food is removed, the therapist removes the spoon from the mouth with the same downward pressure and watches for the swallow. If the rise of the larynx cannot be clearly seen, the therapist should feel for complete elevation. Following the initial swallow, the patient should be asked to open the mouth for visual inspection by the therapist to ensure that no food remains in the mouth. If there is residual, the patient should try again to clear the mouth and swallow or spit it out. If this is unsuccessful, the therapist should clear the mouth with a swab to prevent accumulation and choking. Sometimes the patient may have difficulty moving the bolus from its position on the center of the tongue to swallow. If this problem is evident, food may be placed toward the stronger side of the mouth to compensate; the therapist may later initiate further lateralization exercises of the tongue and jaw.

When jelled or pureed foods are well tolerated, an initial trial of thickened liquid may be attempted. Thickened liquids (yogurt, cream soups cooked with less water), thinned purees (hot cereal with milk or water added), or thick drinks (frappes, nectars) may be chosen. Those items eaten with spoons are administered in the same manner as described. Drinks can be offered in a full shallow cup. To discourage tilting the head back during drinking, a cup with nose cut-out can be used (Figure 6.3); the cut-out faces away from the mouth during drinking. The cup should rest on the lower lip and be tilted to the point at which the liquid touches the upper lip. This encourages mouth closure and allows the patient to sip the liquid actively. Liquid should never be poured into the mouth; nor should the cup be removed after every sip (Mueller, 1975).

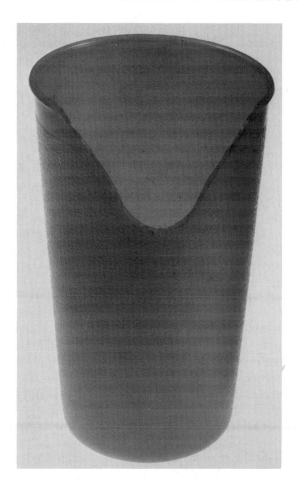

Figure 6.3. Example of a nose cut-out glass to avoid posterior head tilting while drinking. Reprinted by permission of Fred Sammons, Inc.

Initial chewing foods should be soft but not crumbly. Canned fruit cut into small pieces, soft cooked vegetables, and macaroni (sticky) are good choices. Lateral placement of the food in the mouth may initially be needed to position the food for chewing. Facilitation techniques for new skills such as chewing can accompany initial feeding efforts. If early attempts at chewing are weak, the masseter muscles may be vibrated manually during the activity.

Verbal cues or instructions by the therapist may not be needed. If they are indicated because of confusion, hesitation, or difficulty on the part of the patient, they should be brief, concrete, and to the point. ("Would you like Jello? Open your mouth. Close your mouth and take the food. Swallow.") If swallowing difficulty is observed (e.g., the larynx rises but not through the full excursion), more specific instructions can be offered ("Close your mouth. Press your tongue against the roof of your mouth, hold your breath, and swallow.") Some clinicians feel that such actions should be subcortically induced through the appropriate facilitation techniques; however, Griffin (1974) reports successful results training at a cortical level through verbal commands.

Some patients with pseudobulbar dysphagia exhibit signs of inattention, distractability, motor impersistence (inability to sustain an action such as opening the eyes for more than a moment), poor sequencing of the activity, poor judgment, perseveration, and neglect. As a result, they may talk while eating, forget to swallow, overfill the mouth with large spoonfuls of food one after the other, drop food from the mouth, or leave it stored in the mouth long after the meal has ended. In addition to being unappealing, such behavior is dangerous and can lead to aspiration. These patients often respond well to verbal directions that sequence the action and remind them to swallow. There may not be any carryover or improved performance, however, and patients may require careful supervision and verbal cues indefinitely.

The first feeding session should be conservative. Food should be administered slowly, signs of distress monitored, and small amounts of food given. The patient may begin the session with gusto but become suddenly drowsy or less alert. If attempts at sustained arousal fail, the session should be terminated immediately and praise given for the patient's efforts. Despite sensations of hunger, the patient should not expect to eat a full meal and would probably not tolerate one. This may take days or weeks to accomplish.

Following the feeding session, the mouth should be properly cleaned. Lemon-glycerine swabs may be used following each feeding session. The mouth should be checked for any remaining food. If the patient cannot swallow or spit out the residual, it should be promptly removed with a swab, washcloth, or suction catheter. Food should never be washed down with a drink. Swallowing should only proceed in a controlled manner. The soft diet with which neurogenic dysphagics begin training (or on which they remain, especially in the absence of teeth or dentures) can promote growth of bacteria in the mouth. Regular brushing or cleansing of the oral cavity and dentures will help to reduce this.

Finally, the patient should remain in an upright or semiupright position for at least 15 to 30 minutes following the session. This is a precaution against regurgitation or aspiration of food particles remaining in the oral cavity.

APRAXIA

For our purposes, apraxia is defined as inability to perform an intended action at will or to execute an act on command when no significant motor weakness is present. Apraxia can interfere with attempts the patient makes at self-feeding and is often misinterpreted as unwillingness to cooperate. Thus we may choose to address the activity at a subcortical rather than cortical level. For example, if the therapist asks an apraxic patient to blow, an initial awkward and ineffectual attempt might be made, followed by a quizzical shrug of the shoulders as the patient gives up. If the therapist strikes a match and holds it in front of the patient's lips, however, the patient may automatically blow out the match without thinking much about it. The trick is to appeal to this level of subcortical response. Since this book addresses the adult patient, we are talking about an individual who has had a lifetime of habits and routines. Like the global aphasic, the apraxic patient will always perform best an activity that makes use of familiar habits. Following are suggestions for application of feeding training:

1.   The training session should be structured as naturally as possible by positioning the patient in a chair and setting the table with the usual utensils and food items. Distractions such as extraneous food or feeding equipment must be avoided.
2.   Lengthy explanations and instructions that will bring the activity to a cortical level are to be avoided. Rather, the session can be introduced briefly with a cue to help initiate the task: "I've brought your lunch. Would you like a spoon to eat your fruit?", then handing the spoon to the patient.
3.   If the patient seems unable to initiate the task, the starting action can be provided by the therapist by placing the spoon into the dish and ready to scoop, or scooping a small amount of food into the spoon and then offering it to the patient to take.
4.   Some apraxias are restricted to the actions of an involved arm (limb apraxia). In this case, the difficulty may be alleviated by feeding the patient initially, thereby not calling on the apraxic limb.
5.   Oral apraxia is restricted to lip, mouth, and tongue actions. In this case, one can delay testing oral functions purely by command and elicit the same responses by other means. For example, instead of asking the patient to stick out the tongue or move it side to side, one can present a lollipop to lick (useful in inducing a spontaneous swallow), apply a bit of jelly to the lip to lick off, or press a tongue blade against the side of the tongue in the mouth to elicit automatic resistance to the movement. Often oral apraxia will not interfere with eating as much as the initiation of eating or self-feeding; once actual food is presented, the patient often knows what to do with it.

USE OF ADAPTIVE EQUIPMENT

The primary goal for the dysphagic patient is to achieve a full oral diet without risk of aspiration. A secondary goal is to increase the level of independence during eating, so that it is possible to eat in customary fashion. Often during the early sessions the trainer may feed the patient the initial test foods to ensure the greatest caution and care in administration of each mouthful and to control feeding to the utmost.

Unless there is severe limb apraxia or other physical disability preventing self-feeding, the alert patient can soon take over. Some disabilities, however, necessitate retraining. For example, a right-handed patient with right-sided paralysis will need to learn to eat with the left hand. Depending on the extent of damage to other functions (e.g., intellectual abilities, vision, perceptual motor functions, and the patient's premorbid abilities with the left hand), this may proceed smoothly or with great difficulty and frustration. There is a wide array of assistive devices available through specialty companies or distributed locally by the major suppliers of medical and rehabilitative equipment. Sometimes a particular design of a common utensil available in supermarkets or department stores will suffice. Occasionally, the family or trainer can adapt a common utensil with a bit of glue or tape. Usually the biggest problem is keeping track of special aids in the hospital or nursing home. The following are examples of common helpful items.

Dishes

For patients with incoordination or awkwardness, ataxia, or visual impairment, there are large-rimmed dishes and plate guards to keep food from sliding off the plates (Figure 6.4). Some are weighted and/or have nonskid bottoms to increase their stability and reduce accidental spillage.

Nonskid Pads

A nonskid pad can be placed under any bowl or plate for stability (Figure 6.5). A wet washcloth or napkin will also perform this function to a lesser degree.

Drinking Cups

For the incoordinated or visually impaired patient, a heavy plastic mug with a handle large enough for the hand to fit through is best. Clear plastic is ideal. Children's training cups have slotted lids to control the amount sipped (or spilled) and some have weighted rounded bottoms that right themselves when tipped. Spouted tops should be avoided as they encourage primitive sucking behavior. A 50-cc syringe can be used similarly to the sucking facilitator described earlier, but in a more passive manner to elicit early swallowing of liquids in tiny amounts. The large syringe tip presses the lips while several drops can be squirted into the mouth by the trainer. Caution must

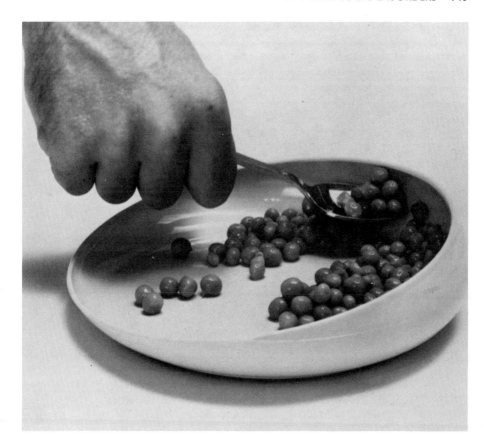

Figure 6.4. Example of a high-scooped dish that assists the patient in loading the utensil for self-feeding. Reprinted by permission of Fred Sammons, Inc.

be used as the squirt can propel liquid unexpectedly to the back of the oral cavity. Long plastic straws available from most prosthetic supply companies can be used by patients who cannot raise a cup to the mouth due to impairments of coordination or weakness. The straws come in varying diameters, rigid or flexible. Rigid straws can be angled by spot-heating with a heat gun. Not all patients relearn sucking adequately, and for some the regular-sized straws require too much sucking strength. Wide plastic straws may ease this problem.

Utensils

There are many varieties of utensils available for impairments of coordination, strength, or range of motion. To assist a weak or poor grip, utensils

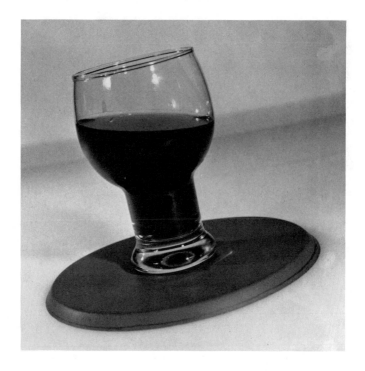

Figure 6.5.   Use of a nonslip rubberized disc for holding eating utensils in place to prevent sliding. Reprinted by permission of Maddak, Inc. Pequannock, NJ.

are designed with large handles. A built-up handle can be made easily by wrapping adhesive tape, a washcloth, plastic tubing, or self-adhesive foam around the handle of a utensil, but these will eventually soil or tear. For long-term use, it is worth purchasing a hard plastic, dishwasher-safe, built-up utensil. For the patient with ataxia or tremors, weighted handles (or weighted wrist cuffs) are available to slow or hold down the affected limb. This is not always effective, especially if there is accompanying weakness. Angled, self-handle, and swivel utensils (Figure 6.6) are available for patients with various limitations in motions. The rocker knife (Figure 6.7) for the one-handed eater cuts meat by a rocking motion instead of the sawing motion that requires holding a fork in another hand. These are sharp utensils and should be avoided if the patient is uncoordinated. The pusher-spoon (see Figure 7.1) or medicine spoon available in some pharmacies has a slide in the handle to push food off into the mouth. This is generally used by the trainer for patients who cannot remove the food from the spoon with their lips or direct it adequately inside the mouth.

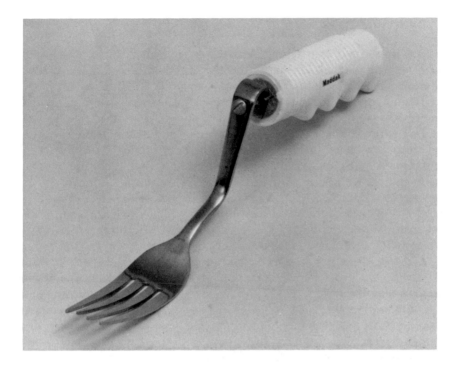

Figure 6.6.   Self-leveling swivel utensil rotates at the handle making feeding easier for patients with limited upper extremity movement. The swivel pin permits the utensil to remain level even though the handle is rotated through an arc of up to 60 degrees. Reprinted by permission of Maddak, Inc. Pequannock, NJ.

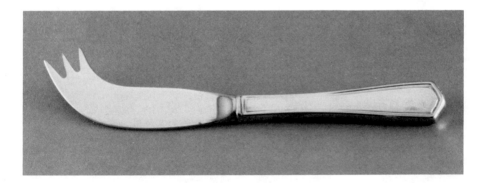

Figure 6.7.   The rocker knife-fork assists the one-handed eater in cutting by using a rocking rather than a sawing motion. Reprinted by permission of Fred Sammons, Inc.

Devices for Major Motor Weakness

Aids are prescribed to maximize independence, not dependence. For that reason, devices are chosen that afford the minimum assistance but still can be handled by the patient. The reason is twofold: first, to use as much of the patient's capabilities as possible, and second, to avoid overequipping the patient with specialized items that can become burdensome.

For extreme hand weakness, the universal cuff is a small and convenient hand strap that has a cuff in the palm that can fit the handle of any regular utensil (Figure 6.8). No hand motion is needed to use it, but the patient or an assistant must slide the cuff on the hand and fit on the utensil.

For large muscle or proximal muscle weakness, the arm can be supported by a wheelchair lap board, ball-bearing feeder (Figure 6.9), or overhead suspension sling (Figure 6.10) that supports the forearm. It requires some muscle power, however poor, to bring the arm from food to mouth.

Electronic devices are not covered here as they require specially trained personnel to analyze the need, prescribe, and assist the severely handicapped patient in their use. All of these adaptive feeding aids are best recommended by an occupational therapist trained in evaluating, prescribing, and educating the patient. All dysphagia team members, however, should be aware of the potential of each patient for self-feeding and know what can be done to maximize these strengths with adaptive equipment.

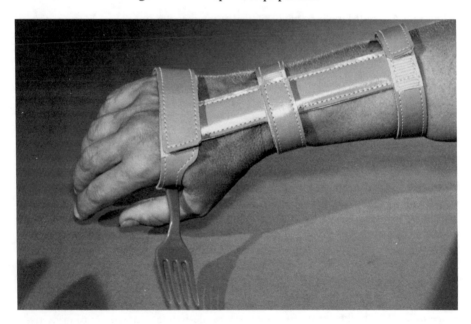

Figure 6.8. The universal cuff fits over the patient's hand, pictured here with a wrist support splint; it requires only arm motion for feeding. Reprinted by permission of Fred Sammons, Inc.

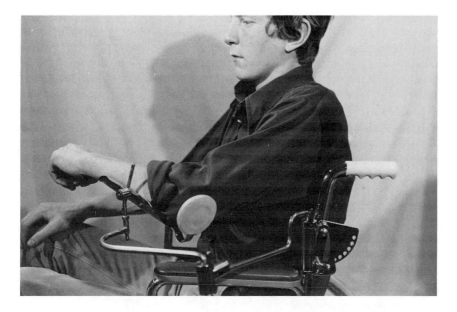

Figure 6.9.   The Michigan feeder is useful for patients with large muscle or proximal weakness. Reprinted by permission of the publisher, from Trombly and Scott, *Occupational therapy for physical dysfunction.* Baltimore: Williams & Wilkins, © 1977. Photographer: Judith LaDrew.

SUMMARY

This chapter provides the clinician with suggestions relating specifically to the first feeding session with the neurologically dysphagic patient following the diagnostic evaluation. Feeding techniques discussed in this chapter should not be overgeneralized. Their application must be individualized. This first feeding encounter needs to be well planned, and the execution must take advantage of the patient's neurologic strengths. These strengths must be nurtured, and in some cases altered to the patient's best advantage. Clinician-imposed controls such as maintaining a distraction-free environment play an equally important role. Prefeeding remediation such as neurofacilitation and/or inhibition may require particular attention. Diet selection and appropriate modifications must be considered if the patient is to succeed with oral intake. A thorough understanding of the general treatment guidelines as presented in Chapter 5 will enable a therapist to begin formulating some treatment rationales for oral feeding of the neurologically compromised patient.

REFERENCES

Ayres AJ. Sensory integration and learning disorders. Los Angeles: Western Psychological Services, 1973.

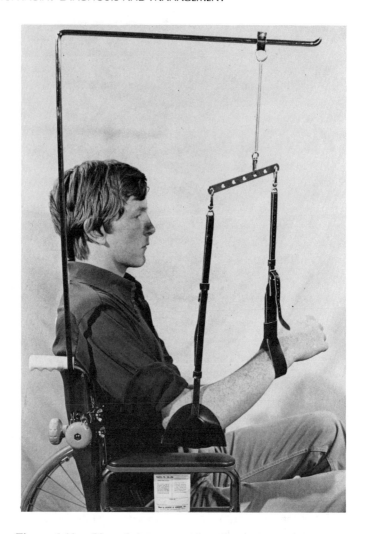

Figure 6.10.   Use of the suspension sling can aid patients in self-feeding. Reprinted by permission of the publisher, from Trombly and Scott, *Occupational therapy for physical dysfunction*. Baltimore: Williams & Wilkins, © 1977. Photographer: Judith LaDrew.

Bosma J, ed. Second symposium on oral sensation and perception. Springfield, Ill.: Charles C Thomas, 1970.

Farber SD. Neurorehabilitation: a multisensory approach. Philadelphia: W B Saunders, 1982.

Fiorentino MR. Reflex testing methods for evaluating CNS development. Springfield, Ill.: Charles C Thomas, 1974.

Griffin KM. Swallowing training for dysphagic patients. Arch Phys Med Rehabil 1974;55:467–70.

Huffman AL. Biofeedback treatment of orofacial dysfunction: a preliminary study. Am J Occup Ther 1978;32:149–54.

Mueller H. Feeding. In: Finnie NR, ed. Handling the young cerebral palsy child at home. New York: C P Dutton, 1975.

Silverman EH, Elfant IL. Dysphagia: an evaluation and treatment program for the adult. Am J Occup Ther 1979;33:382–92.

Trombly CA, Scott AD. Occupational therapy for physical dysfunction. Baltimore: Williams & Wilkins, 1977.

CHAPTER 7

Treatment of Mechanical Swallowing Disorders
Susan M. Fleming

The problems associated with mechanical dysphagia are multifaceted and may cause an array of management possibilities. Thus determining the optimal plan can be challenging. A traditional means of discussing deglutition is to refer to the oropharyngeal and esophageal stages of swallowing. This chapter uses that classification system. Some clarification of problems associated with dysphagia is provided to establish a clearer concept of management guidelines. This is followed by suggestions for treating patients with difficulties of bolus transport during the first two stages of swallowing.

DESCRIPTION OF DISORDERS

Generally, dysphagia involves problems of bolus transport, aspiration, or components of both.

Aspiration is of greatest concern since it is life threatening. At one time or another, most people have aspirated food or liquid into their airway. In healthy persons this results in a cough to expel the substance. In dysphagic patients whose overall physical status may be deteriorated, aspiration may be tolerated poorly.

Aspiration may be caused by unilateral incompetence of the hypoglossal nerve. In this circumstance the process of swallowing is out of control, the tongue no longer able to regulate the passage of the bolus. The pharynx receives the bolus prematurely, threatening the unprotected airway. Considering also that the laryngeal elevators may be impaired with hypoglossal nerve dysfunction, care must be taken in assessing potential risk of aspiration. In other words, disruption of tongue control is not the only factor in hypoglossal nerve dysfunction.

Involvement of the soft palate alone does not result in aspiration. In many neurologic disorders, however, problems of the soft palate accompany problems of the pharynx because of common innervation by the vagus and glossopharyngeal nerves. If peristalsis is disrupted, aspiration is possible since swallowing is such a rapid, synchronous process. Bolus stasis in the pharynx indicates that once the structures assume an at-rest or nonswallowing position, food may enter the unprotected airway. Further down the alimentary tract, a stricture of the cricopharyngeus or upper esophagus could result in regurgitation of swallowed substance that might then be spilled into the unprotected airway.

Problems of bolus transport can occur anywhere along the feeding route. For example, a person with unilateral involvement of the hypoglossal nerve with resection of portions of the tongue would have difficulty lateralizing a bolus for mastication and transport into the oropharynx to initiate the second stage of swallowing. Resection or paralysis of the soft palate may result in nasal regurgitation of the bolus, especially if the bolus is liquid (Kilman and Goyal, 1976). Pharyngeal involvement results in disrupted peristaltic activity of the pharyngeal constrictors. Stenosis or narrowing of the alimentary tract at the level of the cricopharyngeus may prevent a food bolus from moving beyond that point. Esophageal transit may be disrupted in a similar manner.

Prior to deciding which mechanical devices to use in aiding bolus transport, the clinician must have medicolegal clearance to work with the dysphagic patient. Presuming legal consent such as clinical privileges and medical clearance have been obtained, the clinician must completely review the patient's chart as a beginning to a thorough assessment. If the patient appears to be at risk for aspiration (e.g., frequently coughs, has a "wet" sounding voice, or is unable to clear secretions well), the clinician must discuss this with the attending physician. Assuming that the patient is not at significant risk of aspiration, mechanical devices can be considered to enable the patient to eat more easily and more conveniently, and most importantly, to maintain nutrition and hydration.

FEEDING DEVICES

Glossectomy Feeding Spoons

Glossectomy feeding spoons provide a means of transporting the bolus of food to the oropharynx. Not all patients with a partial or total glossectomy are candidates for the device. There are two criteria for use of the spoon. First, the patient should not be considered a high risk for aspiration. Significant resection of the base of the tongue or problems at the pharyngeal stage of swallowing might render the larynx vulnerable to the oncoming bolus. In addition, swallowing may be compromised severely in patients with resection of the hyomandibular complex (Summers, 1971). Second, the patient can use the glossectomy feeding spoon with greatest ease if at least 50 percent of the tongue has been resected. The presence of more tongue actually interferes with placement of the device.

Pureed (blenderized) or finely chopped food is placed in the bowl of the spoon. The food should be ground to a consistency that eliminates the need for mastication. If lubrication is a problem, gravies, juices, and the like can be mixed in with the food. Holding the spoon level to keep the bolus from falling off, the bowl is placed as far back into the oral cavity as possible (avoid eliciting a gag reflex). Placement should be on the side where the patient has greater tongue mass remaining and/or better sensation. Sliding the triggering mechanism on the handle will cause the push plate on the bowl of the spoon to move and deposit the food onto the base of the tongue.

The glossectomy feeding spoon is useful because it gives patients an opportunity to enjoy something besides liquids that are transported by way of other devices. It is also more esthetically acceptable than a tube since it closely resembles commonly used flatware. There are at least two types of metal glossectomy feeding spoons available today (Figure 7.1). The one shown on the bottom of the figure is available to eligible military veterans through the prosthetics center of the Veterans Administration. Developed at the VA Medical Center, Allen Park, Michigan, the device has been used by several patients and found quite acceptable. The spoon shown at the top of Figure 7.1 is available commercially through Fred Sammons, Inc., Brook-

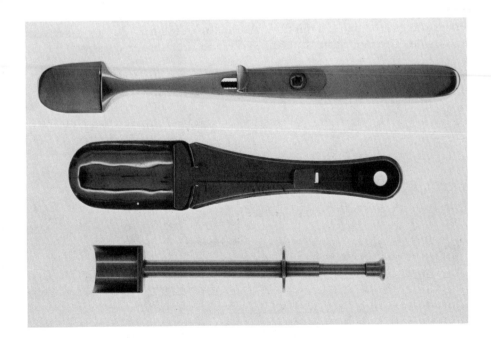

Figure 7.1.   (Top) Commercially available glossectomy feeding spoon. (Middle) Cooking measuring spoon that should not be used for feeding. (Bottom) Glossectomy feeding spoon available for eligible military veterans.

field, Illinois. Shown in the middle of Figure 7.1 is a measuring spoon used for cooking. It is included here only to show what should not be used for feeding patients; other than being somewhat unwieldly, it is risky to use, as the push plate easily slides out from the spoon's handle and may be inadvertently deposited into the patient's oropharynx.

If the patient is not an eligible military veteran, or if funding is not available to purchase the commercially available spoon, a glossectomy feeding spoon can be constructed readily by the clinician (Fleming and Weaver, 1983). It may not be as esthetically pleasing or as easy to use (particularly if trismus is present) as the one described, but it will be economical and based on the same principles. It is made from a 20-cc plastic syringe (Figure 7.2). Using a medium-fine hacksaw blade, a horizontal cut is made to one side of the protruding tip at the distal end of the syringe. A second cut is made perpendicular to the first cut so that the larger portion of the distal tip may be removed and discarded. A beveled 45 degree third cut is made on the cylinder wall about 3 cm from the distal end of the cylinder. This cut should continue only to the midpoint of the cylinder. Finally, two parallel cuts are made into the cylinder from the distal end toward the proximal end, intercepting the third cut. The portion of the cylinder that is sectioned by the third and fourth cuts is discarded. The inner portion of the cylinder is then ground down enough so that the piston can move freely. Fine sandpaper is used to remove bits of plastic and to smooth rough edges. The entire process takes less than ten minutes. At the top of Figure 7.3 is a glossectomy feeding device made from a plastic syringe in the manner described.

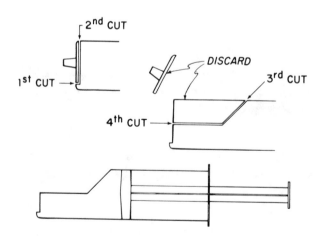

Figure 7.2.   Steps used in making a glossectomy feeding spoon from a 20-cc plastic syringe. See the top of Figure 7.3 for the finished product.

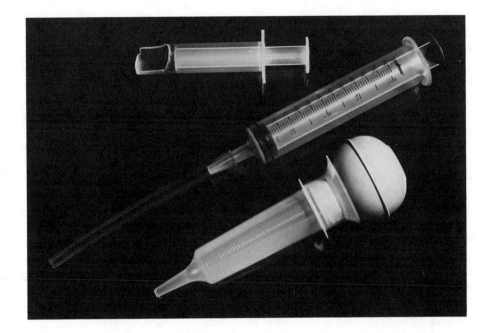

Figure 7.3.   (Top) Glossectomy feeding spoon made from a 20-cc plastic syringe. (Middle) Catheter-tipped 60-cc syringe with tubular extension device for feeding. (Bottom) Bulb type syringe sometimes used for feeding.

Syringes

Patients with lingual paresis or those having less than 50 percent tongue resection also may have difficulty with transport of an oral bolus. For them, use of the glossectomy feeding spoon is impractical because of the presence of tongue mass. For these patients, a 50- or 60-cc catheter-tipped syringe (Bakamjian and Cramer, 1960) with a 15-cm extension of pliable connecting tubing can be used (Figure 7.3, middle). The syringes can be made of glass, but they are more expensive (approximately 24 dollars each) and more easily broken than the plastic ones. They do have advantages, however, in that they are easy to clean and pistons slide easily within them. Plastic syringes are more difficult to keep clean and the washerlike tip at the distal end of the piston demonstrates wear by sticking, particularly if very warm foods are used. The major advantages of the plastic syringes are that they cost about one-twentieth the amount of the glass syringes and they are unbreakable. Individual circumstances suggest which type of syringe to use, but in most settings it is probably better to start with a plastic model and progress to a glass one when the patient is able to manage the device handily.

Prior to issuing a catheter-tipped syringe with a tubular extension, the risk of aspiration must be considered. Again, it is incumbent upon the clinician to obtain medical clearance before attempting to use the device with a patient. In addition, the clinician must consider the patient's overall ability to handle the syringe. For example, although only a few patients manage syringe feedings with only one hand, the majority require use of both hands (one to support the device and the other to regulate the piston). The bottom of Figure 7.3 shows a bulb type syringe. Most patients find this difficult to control, complaining that it squirts food into their mouths, resulting in a startle or recoil response.

The patient must fill the catheter-tipped syringe by slowly withdrawing the piston as the distal tip of the tubular extension is submerged into a liquid or thin puree. The object is to fill the syringe with food, but not pockets of air. Practice enables most patients to acquire this skill within the first session. To make the task easier, the puree should be strained and not too thick. Once the syringe is filled with food, the patient places the distal tip of the tubular extension at the place in the mouth where there is greatest sensation and ability to move the bolus with the tongue. For patients with surgical excision this is usually on the back of the unresected portion of tongue. For those with cerebrovascular accident or other neuromuscular problem, the distal tip should be placed where the bolus can be most easily handled.

Connecting tubing is the most convenient tubular extension to use since it is available in most settings and its large diameter (approximately 6 mm or 18 French) allows pureed foods to pass. Smaller-diameter tubing (e.g., 3 mm or 10 French) may have at least two applications. First, it allows more precise placement, which is beneficial in stimulation exercises. Second, some patients, such as those with severe trismus, may be unable to open their mouths wide enough for even the 6-mm connecting tube extension. For them a narrower tube may be more easily tolerated.

Finally, there are those patients who, through trauma or elective surgery, must have their teeth wired to prevent jaw opening. For them the problem is usually only a mechanical one—getting liquid food into the oral cavity. A small-gauge feeding tube can be threaded behind the third molar into the oral cavity. Feeding may then proceed with syringe or gavage bag, that is, the pliable plastic container used to hold the tube feeding, commonly referred to as the feeding bag. The attending physician must be informed of intended method of feeding and be assured that the patient can handle the feedings without aspiration.

The optimal position for feeding dysphagic patients is upright, with head support if necessary (Buckley, Addicks, and Maniglia, 1976). The head should not be tilted back, as such a posture only increases the chances of aspiration. The one exception to the upright position is when the patient has a problem transporting an oral bolus compounded by drooling and intraoral pooling, but does not have significant risk of aspiration. Eating may be easier if the patient assumes a semireclining position (e.g., 50 degrees), but with the head and body on the same plane. The goal is to decrease aspiration (head remains on plane with the body, not tilted) while increasing oral transport of the bolus (gravity helps the patient move the bolus to the oropharynx).

The patient with a supraglottic laryngectomy should not extend the head posteriorly in an effort to swallow. There is no reason to do so since transport of the bolus is not a problem. Extending the head posteriorly only increases aspiration because the laryngeal inlet becomes more accessible to the oncoming bolus.

Sometimes it is necessary to remind or train these patients to inhale, swallow, exhale, and reswallow. This sequence of events is almost normal and should be reinforced since it serves to protect the airway and to clear pooled food from the laryngeal aditus. There are two points to emphasize when teaching this normal sequence of inhale, swallow, and exhale. First, exhalation, not inhalation, must follow the swallow. If one were to inhale immediately following a swallow, aspiration would probably occur. Second, the swallow must occur at the beginning, not the end, of the exhalation phase of respiration. This allows an adequate amount of pulmonary air to help clear the laryngeal aditus. Another swallow must follow to clear any materials pooled in the pharyngeal recesses.

Nasogastric Tubes

Unfortunately, in spite of efforts to rehabilitate dysphagic patients, there are times that adequate oral nutrition and hydration are not possible. Although problems associated with patients handling their own secretions persist, those problems associated with aspiration of food and fluids can be circumvented through other means. Surgically, an altered feeding route, such as a feeding gastrostoma or esophagostoma, can be created. These procedures are reserved for patients whose eating problems are considered long term (see Chapter 10). Parenteral feeding is one method of supplying nutrition (Hegedus and Pelham, 1975) (see Chapter 9). Another option is the use of a nasogastric (NG) feeding tube (Figure 7.4). Although feeding tubes come with a variety of features, perhaps the most important one is their diameter. From the standpoint of patient comfort and fewer complications, the smaller size (10 French) is preferred; it also achieves a slower rate of feeding. Patients with larger feeding tubes (16 to 18 French) tend to feed themselves too rapidly, which causes gastric distress (Cataldo and Smith, 1980). Also, esophageal ulceration increases with larger tubes, especially if they are employed for an extended period of time. The only advantages to larger feeding tubes are that they are easier to insert and do not clog as easily as the smaller ones. (See Chapter 9 for additional discussion of NG tubes.) These are staff conveniences that do not necessarily improve the patient's comfort and tolerance.

For patients who abhor the thought of being seen outside the hospital setting with a nasogastric feeding tube in place, there is an alternative. They

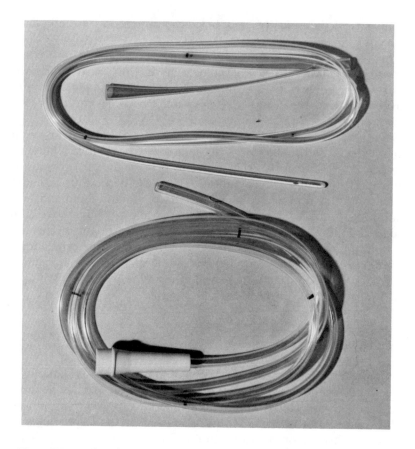

Figure 7.4. (Top) Small (10 French) nasogastric feeding tube. (Bottom) Large (16 French) nasogastric feeding tube.

can be taught to carefully insert a shorter feeding tube, take the feeding, withdraw the tube, and clean it properly after use (Donaldson, Skelly, and Paletta, 1968) (Figure 7.5). If they so desire, they can become accustomed to the procedure. The obvious risk is, of course, incorrect insertion of the tube. The objective is to place the distal tip of the reusable tube into the upper esophagus so that it bypasses the level of the pharynx where food might be aspirated into the larynx. The decision to use this device rests with the physician and dysphagia team members and is based on their perception of how adequately the patient can adapt to the method.

TRACHEOSTOMA TUBES

Many patients with mechanical dysphagia have a tracheostoma tube in place, especially in the acute stage of their illness. While tracheostoma tubes assure

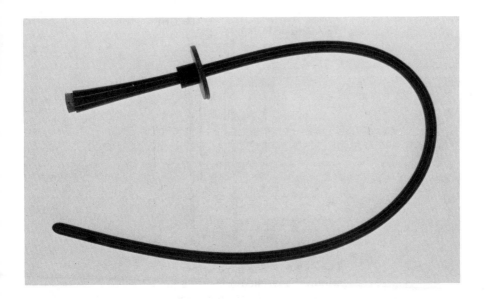

Figure 7.5.   Nasoesophageal feeding tube with safety retention flange.

an airway, they do interfere with swallowing. In a retrospective study, Arms, Dines, and Tinstman (1974) demonstrated increased risk of aspiration with their presence. Normally, when one swallows, the larynx is lifted in an anterosuperior direction to protect the laryngeal inlet from the oncoming bolus. The presence of a tracheostoma tube may anchor the larynx and make it more accessible to the bolus (Bonanno, 1971). Another problem concerns pulmonary air, which cannot be used to clear the larynx if obstructions impede the flow of air. Normally, immediately following a swallow we exhale to clear the laryngeal aditus of foreign substance. With a tracheostoma tube, pulmonary air is shunted out via the tube. Figure 7.6 illustrates how most of the pulmonary air is shunted out of the tracheostoma tube when the outer cannula takes up such a large portion of the inner diameter of the trachea. The usual manner of clearing the larynx is not available. Nothing can be done about the presence of the tracheostoma tube limiting anterosuperior laryngeal elevation, but there are some things to consider about improving the flow of pulmonary air through the larynx.

The most practical way to effect passage of air through the larynx instead of out the tracheostoma tube itself is to plug or cover the opening of the tube. The patient can do this with the index finger, which is effective for the immediate purpose, but it is not convenient since it necessitates the continued use of one hand. Full closure plugs (Figure 7.7) can be used to occlude the port. These (Pilling Co.) are tapered and fitted by size so that there is no danger of their being drawn into the trachea. Another means of closing the opening of the tracheostoma tube is by use of a one-way Kistner

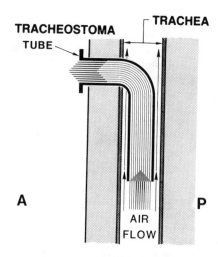

Figure 7.6. The large arrow within the tracheostoma tube indicates a significant proportion of air shunted out of the tracheostoma tube. Smaller arrows show a relatively small proportion of pulmonary air available for clearing the laryngeal aditus.

valve (Figure 7.8). The Kistner valve opens on inhalation and closes when the user exhales. Exhaled air passes upward through the larynx. It should be noted that if a tracheostoma tube diameter is so large that it occludes much of the inner tracheal diameter, no amount of plugging at the open end of the tube will allow pulmonary air to reach the larynx. This is a mechanical blockage that must be dealt with. The simplest solution is to reduce the tracheostoma tube by two sizes. For example, if a patient with a number 8 tube cannot get adequate air to the larynx for phonation or coughing when the tracheostoma opening is plugged, a number 6 tube should be used.

Another way to get pulmonary air to pass upward into the larynx is by use of a fenestrated tracheostoma tube (Figure 7.9, top). Some of these also are provided with a valve for the fenestration. These work well unless the patient has copious secretions that could impede the functioning of the fenestration and its valve. Their use may be limited because of problems associated with irritation of the tracheal wall. To eliminate this irritation no part of the fenestration should be adjacent to the tracheal wall. Verification of fenestration location may be done radiographically.

Cuffed tracheostoma tubes present problems such as infection, tracheal stenosis, esophageal erosion, and innominate artery fistualization (Cooper and Grillo, 1969; Sasaki, 1980). The cuff is inflated to keep food, liquid, and secretions from getting into the lungs. The top of Figure 7.10 shows a cuff that is inflated; the cuff in the bottom of the figure is not inflated. The

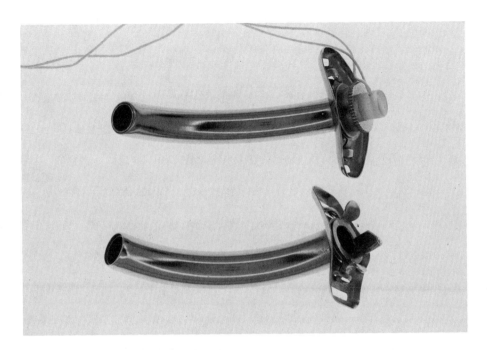

Figure 7.7. (Top) Full closure plugs can be used to occlude the tracheostoma. (Bottom) Unplugged tracheostoma tube.

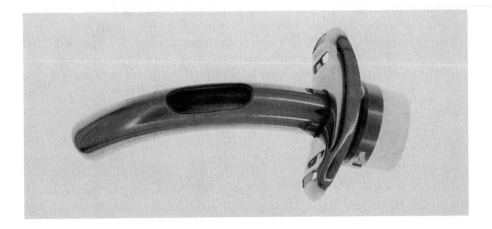

Figure 7.8. A one-way valved tracheostoma tube.

cuff should be inflated to the specifications of the physician (Nahum and Harris, 1981).

There are, however, three reasons for not feeding patients orally while their tracheostoma cuffs are inflated. First, if a patient's medical condition

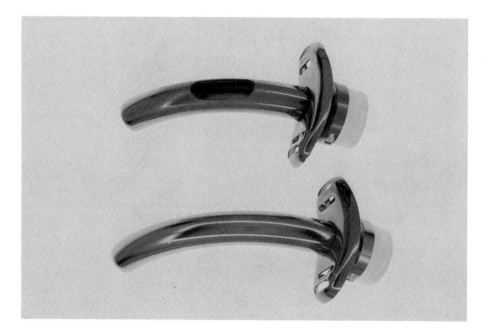

Figure 7.9.   (Top) Fenestrated and one-way valved tracheostoma tube. (Bottom) Unfenestrated and one-way valved tracheostoma tube.

is so precarious that a cuffed tracheostoma tube is warranted, perhaps oral feeding is premature. It has been demonstrated radiographically that a liquid bolus may get past the cuff and enter the lower trachea. Second, presence of an inflated cuff prevents pulmonary air from clearing the larynx; this mechanical blockage is not desirable. Third, if a patient is aspirating the food bolus it is vital to know when it occurs so that suctioning can be done immediately. With an inflated cuff that knowledge is delayed.

There are guidelines for working with these patients. Once medical clearance has been obtained, the tracheostoma should be suctioned, the cuff deflated, and suctioning repeated. Then the patients may be fed. Adding a bit of food coloring to the food will help verify aspiration. Once the patients have been fed they should be suctioned again and the cuff inflated to the physician's specifications.

SYNTHETIC SALIVA

Patients taking certain medications and those patients receiving irradiation to the oral or pharyngeal areas will experience xerostomia or dry mouth

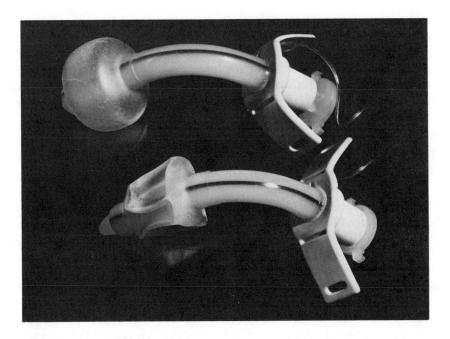

Figure 7.10.   (Top) Cuffed tracheostoma tube with cuff inflated. (Bottom) Cuffed tracheostoma tube with cuff somewhat deflated.

(Shedd, 1976; Dreizen et al., 1977; Sobol, Conoyer, and Sessions, 1979). In addition to physical discomfort, this causes at least two other problems. First, there is the loss of saliva that normally serves to cleanse and protect the teeth. Without the protection provided by saliva, dental caries increase (Trowbridge and Carl, 1975). Second, with decreased saliva there is reduction in the ability to moisten food and facilitate mastication and deglutition (Mansson and Sandberg, 1975). This leads to weight loss in many patients.

Although saliva cannot be replaced, artificial saliva is available to provide lubrication. Two products available through the Veterans Administration are Artificial Saliva #80 and VA-Oralube. Two products commercially available are Moi-Stir (Kingswood Laboratories) and Salivart (Westport Pharmaceuticals). Usually patients are directed to take the synthetic saliva as needed. Most rinse with a spoonful of the synthetic saliva just prior to eating. Some of these products contain fluoride needed to deter caries formation (Dudgeon, DeLisa, and Miller, 1980). Unfortunately, some may have a drying effect (Daeffler, 1981); therefore their use must be assessed on an individual basis.

Lemon-glycerin swabs are available for the patient to cleanse and freshen the mouth. Although for many patients these special swabs provide relief, others find that they add to oral dryness with long-term use. Thus patient preference will help determine the amount and frequency of use of lemon-glycerin swabs.

In addition to synthetic saliva, a surface anesthetic applied just prior to eating may help reduce the pain associated with deglutition. Surface anesthesia should be used carefully in those patients at high risk for aspiration, since the swallowing mechanism should not be further compromised by reduced sensation.

FOOD BLENDERS

Perhaps the most a clinician can do for the patient is to provide the food consistency that is best tolerated. Unfortunately, most people assume that liquid consistency is best. This is not necessarily so. Many patients with mechanical disorders leading to dysphagia do better with food of puree consistency (Ardran and Kemp, 1952; Summers, 1971; Edwards, 1973; Paavolainen, 1977; Silverman and Elfant, 1979). Pureed material is less mobile than liquid, and with an impaired oropharyngeal mechanism it is important to minimize aspiration. This is especially true of the patient who has undergone a supraglottic laryngectomy. Evidence of this is supported by our clinical experience and radiographic observations. Fluids are more easily tolerated by patients who demonstrate an organic stenosis (Hellemans, Pelemans, and Vantrappen, 1981).

Food consistency is of such importance that some facilities make food blenders available to patients. An added benefit of blenders is that the cost of purchasing specially prepared products can be reduced as patients are able to puree items that are consumed by the rest of the family (Farrior and Kelly, 1979).

SUMMARY

Mechanical swallowing disorders in the mouth, pharynx, and esophagus usually result from a combination of structure loss and/or rearrangement and potential peripheral nerve involvement secondary to removal of cancerous lesions. Such lesions in the mouth and pharynx may require glossectomy, partial pharyngectomy, and partial laryngectomy resulting in difficulty transporting and channeling a bolus. Decisions concerning the appropriate mechanical device and diet needed to obviate mechanical disorders are based on the type and amount of resection, concomitant medical complications, and patient acceptance and cooperation. Alternatives to regular dietary intake via nasogastric tube feeding, surgically created feeding routes, and blenderized textures need to be considered.

REFERENCES

Ardran GM, Kemp FH. The protection of the laryngeal airway during swallowing. Br J Radiol 1952;23:406–16.

Arms RA, Dines DE, Tinstman TC. Aspiration pneumonia. Chest 1974;65:136–39.

Bakamjian V, Cramer L. Surgical management of advanced cancer of the tongue. Ann Surg 1960;152:1058–66.

Bonanno PC. Swallowing dysfunction after tracheostomy. Ann Surg 1971;174:29–33.

Buckley JE, Addicks CL, Maniglia J. Feeding patients with dysphagia. Nurs Forum 1976;15:69–85.

Cataldo CB, Smith L. Tube feedings: clinical applications. Columbus, Ohio: Ross Laboratories, 1980.

Cooper JD, Grillo HC. The evolution of tracheal injury due to ventilatory assistance through cuffed tubes: a pathologic study. Ann Surg 1969;169:334–48.

Daeffler R. Oral hygiene measures for patients with cancer. Cancer Nurs 1981;4:29–35.

Donaldson RC, Skelly M, Paletta FX. Total glossectomy for cancer. Am J Surg 1968;116:585–90.

Dreizen S, Daly TE, Drane JB, Brown LR. Oral complications of cancer radiotherapy. Postgrad Med 1977;61:85–92.

Dudgeon BJ, DeLisa JA, Miller RM. Head and neck cancer, a rehabilitation approach. Am J Occup Ther 1980;34:243–51.

Edwards H. Neurological disease of the pharynx and larynx. Practitioner 1973; 211:729–37.

Farrior JB III, Kelly MT. Home nutrition for patients with head and neck tumors. Ear Nose Throat J 1979;58:84–85.

Fleming SM, Weaver AW. Glossectomy feeding device readily adapted from a plastic syringe. Arch Phys Med Rehabil 1983;64:183–5.

Hegedus S, Pelham M. Dietetics in a cancer hospital. J Am Diet Assoc 1975;67:235–40.

Hellemans J, Pelemans W, Vantrappen G. Pharyngoesophageal swallowing disorders and the pharyngo-esophageal sphincter. Med Clin North Am 1981;65:1149–71.

Kilman WJ, Goyal RK. Disorders of pharyngeal and upper esophageal sphincter motor function. Arch Intern Med 1976;136:592–601.

Mansson I, Sandberg N. Salivary stimulus and swallowing reflex in man. Acta Otolaryngol 1975;79:445–50.

Nahum AM, Harris JP, Davidson TM. The patient who aspirates—diagnosis and management. J Otolaryngol 1981;10:10–16.

Paavolainen M. Rehabilitation of eating after supraglottic laryngectomy. Minerva Otorhinolaryngol 1977;27:91–5.

Sasaki CT. Paralysis of the larynx and pharynx. Surg Clin North Am 1980;60:1079–92.

Shedd DP. Rehabilitation problems of head and neck cancer patients. J Surg Oncol 1976;8:11–21.

Silverman EH, Elfant IL. Dysphagia: an evaluation and treatment program for the adult. Am J Occup Ther 1979;33:382–92.

Sobol SM, Conoyer JM, Sessions DG. Enteral and parenteral nutrition in patients with head and neck cancer. Ann Otolaryngol 1979;88:495–501.

Summers GW. Physiologic problems following ablative surgery of the head and neck. Otolaryngol Clin North Am 1971;7:217–50.

Trowbridge JE, Carl W. Oral care of the patient having head and neck irradiation. Am J Nurs 1975;75:2146–49.

PART III

Supportive and Alternative Management Approaches to Deglutitory Dysfunction

CHAPTER 8

Nutritional Considerations
Abby S. Bloch

Adequate nutrition is frequently overlooked or neglected as a component of management in the dysphagic patient. Studies conducted at various medical centers supported the existing belief of clinicians working in clinical nutrition that patients become more malnourished the longer they remain in the hospital (Allardyce and Groves, 1974; Bistrian et al., 1976; Shils, 1981). Responsible nutrition management must be provided for all patients, but those with dysphagia are at increased risk due to their physical limitations as well as physiologic and emotional components. As patients become more and more malnourished, they lose the ability to digest and use foodstuffs. As intake of calories and protein decrease below requirements, the body becomes unable to generate intestinal epithelium lining cells. The villi and microvilli needed to metabolize and absorb foods flatten and become ineffective, leading to malabsorption. Attention to appropriate nutrition support will provide improved care for these patients.

ASSESSING THE PATIENT'S STATUS

Patients who are nutritionally at risk or potentially at risk must be identified so that they can be given appropriate therapy. This can be done by a simple assessment that is part of an in-depth work-up form or a separate questionnaire (Bloch, 1980) (Figure 8.1). Any member of the clinical care team (intern, resident, dietitian, or nurse) may collect the data.

---

1. a. What is your usual weight? _____pounds
   b. What is your height? _____feet _____inches
   c. Have you gained weight? no_____ yes_____
      If yes, how many pounds? _____ Have you lost weight? no_____
      yes_____ *If yes,* how many pounds? _____Over what period of time? _____
2. Is your present appetite usual? _____better? _____worse than before your illness?

Figure 8.1. Suggested format for dietary screening assessment.

3. a. Do you have problems related to eating? no_____ yes_____
    If yes, check the appropriate reason(s): sore mouth_____
    swallowing_____ chewing_____ choking_____
    nausea_____ salivation_____ change in taste_____
    food aversion_____ vomiting_____ diarrhea_____
    constipation_____ other_____
   b. How many meals do you eat daily?_____
   c. Do you need help in eating? no_____ yes_____
4. Do you wear dentures? upper_____ lower_____ none_____
5. a. Were you previously on a special diet? no_____ yes_____
    If yes, please check: low sodium_____ low fat_____
    low sugar_____ other_____
   b. Do you take vitamins or minerals? no_____ yes_____
    If yes, please list_____

    c. Do you have any personal or religious dietary restrictions? kosher_____
    vegetarian_____ other (specify):_____

6. Do you have allergies or intolerances for food? no_____ yes_____
   If yes, please list:_____

7. Do you take commercial nutritional supplements? no_____ yes_____
   If yes, please list:_____

DO NOT WRITE BELOW THIS LINE—FOR DIETITIAN'S USE ONLY

Date of initial visit_____
1. Diagnosis:_____

2. Diet Rx_____
   Supplement Rx_____
3. Expected treatment plan: surgery
   RT_____ chemo_____ other_____
4. Abnormal lab data (list):_____

5. Metabolic and other problems:
   diabetes_____ malabsorption_____
   hypertension_____ type_____
   heart disease___ GI obstruction___
   persistent fever_____ partial_____
   alcohol_____
   renal disease_____ GI fistula_____
   liver disease_____
   other_____

6. Present medications_____

7. Ht:_____cm Adm. wt:_____kg
   Avg std._____kg
   Pre-illness wt:_____lb
   _____kg (pre-illness −
   Adm/pre-illness × 100)
8. Anticipated problems due to
   illness or treatment plan?
   no_____ yes_____

9. Edema: site and degree_____
   ascites_____
10. See progress notes for
    assessment and nutritional
    care plan.

    Dietitian:_____
    Date:_____

Figure 8.1. *(continued)*

Based on the hospital's patient population, type of medical or surgical procedures, staffing capabilities, number of beds, and rate of patient turnover, a valid set of guidelines or standards can be developed. This may include specific problems related to dysphagia, for example, patients who can swallow liquid or pureed foods; those who can only handle textured, more solid consistency items; or patients who cannot even swallow saliva. Weight changes or other problems related to food intake also should be included in the initial assessment. An elaborate, extensive work-up using sophisticated equipment and in-depth techniques such as body composition or muscle activity studies may be required or desired. For the majority of patients in most settings, however, a simple, rapid form is more than adequate.

For patients who seem to be stable and give no history of nutritionally related food problems prior to dysphagia, a well-balanced diet in the form and consistency that is most easily managed may be adequate. If the patient has lost a significant amount of weight already, increased nutritional support may be necessary. The health professional who is assuming responsibility for the nutrition evaluation must first determine the cause of depletion. Obviously, inadequate food intake ranks number one on the list of mechanisms of malnutrition of the dysphagic patient; however, the cause of poor food intake may vary considerably (see Chapters 2 and 3).

Fear, anxiety, and depression should not be ignored as additional possible causes of poor food intake. Patients who suspect they may have a serious illness or disease, who are undergoing diagnostic studies to rule out disease, or who are being treated for a disease frequently lose weight. Fear of the consequences of long-term illness such as financial problems, family security, and family attitudes toward the patient's own concerns about survival all affect the ability to maintain adequate nutritional intake.

The patient who has lived alone may not have been able to buy food without assistance or prepare meals alone. Pain, swallowing difficulty, and the effort entailed in consuming foods may prevent an individual from sitting long enough to eat an adequate amount. If no one assists at mealtime, a patient may not be able to cut or mash the foods into small enough pieces, position the head to place it properly in the mouth for swallowing, lift utensils or cups, and sit up or assume a comfortable position. Edentulous patients and those with poorly fitting dentures have additional difficulties. A person may be at risk nutritionally for any of these reasons.

Concern about the side effects or aftereffects of eating may lead to diminished intake. A patient may have a desire to eat and have a good appetite, but find that the item is difficult to swallow or that it will cause pain, cramping, gas, diarrhea, nausea, and/or vomiting soon after it is eaten. Eventually, the patient will decide not to eat although still hungry, so as to avoid the negative effects that may result. For instance, concern about social embarrassment because of flatus or diarrhea becomes a significant problem for many patients who do have such a reaction to food.

Medical and surgical therapy may impair the capability of a patient to eat. Many patients who are taking potentially toxic drugs or receiving therapy such as irradiation find that they are not able to eat adequately or may experience periods when their food intake is limited. In addition, many drugs and medications such as antibiotics, amphetamines, analgesics, diuretics, anticonvulsants, antineoplastic agents, and cardiac glycosides can create nausea, vomiting, diarrhea, and other discomforts. These should not be overlooked as part of the nutritional problems that patients experience. Medications and dosages must always be checked for patients who are having nutritional problems.

Patients may give a history of being anorectic. They are disinterested in food, have a very poor appetite, and are easily satiated. This may result from emotional factors and/or as part of a clinical condition.

SELECTING APPROPRIATE FEEDINGS

When the severity of nutritional depletion is determined and its cause is identified, appropriate nutritional therapeutic procedures may be instituted. The clinician must formulate a regimen that will supply adequate amounts of both calories and protein in an appropriate form. If caloric requirements are not met, ingested protein will be used for energy, not tissue synthesis.

The status of the patient's gastrointestinal tract must be evaluated to determine what if any modifications in nutrients are necessary. Can the patient split intact protein into the peptides and amino acids needed for absorption? Can the patient tolerate the osmotic load of monosaccharides or disaccharides? Is the patient intolerant to fats or need special fat? Is the patient lactose intolerant? Are other nutritionally relevant factors involved?

All electrolytes, vitamins, minerals, and trace elements must be provided in adequate amounts to meet daily requirements. If the patient's condition requires increases in certain electrolytes or trace elements due to loss from drainage or increased demands, those items must be replaced in amounts consistent with needs without causing overhydration or underhydration.

If and when the patient is able to eat, there are several guidelines to follow. Initially, it helps to offer regular familiar foods if the patient is able to tolerate them. This also may include those whose meals or food selections must be modified, such as several (e.g., six) small pureed or blenderized feedings, mechanically soft-textured, bland and low-acid, high-calorie diets, or modifications in specific nutrients. It is always desirable, however, to offer as many foods as possible with which the patient is familiar.

If oral feeding proves unsuccessful, high-calorie liquid supplements or protein liquid drinks can be offered when liquids do not present problems (see Appendix 8.A). Supplements may be in the form of malted milk drinks, if the patient can tolerate lactose and fluid. High-calorie between-meal snacks can be in the form of custard or puddings, quiches, souffles, and soft cheese with mashed fruits.

COMMERCIAL PREPARATIONS

Many commercially prepared drinks and formulas are available for patients who can tolerate liquids better than solids (see Appendix 8.B). These drinks are nutritionally complete and are designed to provide a sufficient number of nutrients and calories if an adequate volume is consumed. Many clinicians order one or two cans of a supplement per day for a patient who is eating poorly or losing weight. Unfortunately, one can of a supplement, even if calorically dense, will not have a significant impact on the patient's overall nutritional status. Most commercial preparations have approximately one calorie per cubic centimeter. Therefore one 8-oz can has 240 calories. Several formulas have a higher caloric ratio, 1.5 calories per cubic centimeter. Even with these products, an 8-oz can will provide an additional 350 calories, not enough to meet daily needs. Cans or containers with appropriate volumes could be left at the bedside or within easy reach in an ice bath or Thermos so that the patient can sip the drink throughout the day. Consumption of the entire amount frequently augments calories from an otherwise inadequate intake to permit the patient to meet daily needs.

When patients cannot or will not eat solids, as is the case with many dysphagic as well as weak, debilitated, depressed, or elderly individuals, nutritionally complete liquid formulas may be an effective method of supplying adequate nutrients orally. With the multitude of commercial, complete, defined formula diets now available, patients can be maintained in good nutritional balance if the proper amounts of nutrients are provided. Oral liquid formulas as the sole source of nutrition are effective for patients who have difficulty in chewing or swallowing solids but are able to take liquids.

Patients who are somewhat underweight and need a low-residue intake in preparation for bowel surgery or for postsurgical recovery might profit from a nutritionally complete liquid diet. Typically, they receive a low-protein diet, clear liquids, or intravenous solutions of glucose and water. All provide limited calories and inadequate protein considering the high requirements at this particular time due to stress and increased metabolic activity. This is particularly true when preoperative or postoperative periods of diminished appetite or intake exceed five days.

Commercial preparations vary in lactose content, residue, and caloric density. To assure tolerance, the correct formulas must be selected. Currently, approximately 35 products are available for enteral use, varying in protein content, type, caloric density, electrolyte concentration, packaging, and cost (Shils, 1977; Shils, Bloch, and Chernoff, 1979). To meet the needs of a given patient, selection must be made based on knowledge and evaluation of each product. Arbitrary decisions can be inappropriate for a given patient.

FEEDING PROBLEMS OF HOSPITALIZED PATIENTS

Hospitalized patients may have problems achieving adequate nutritional intake for reasons other than dysphagia. Anxiety and emotional reactions to the hospital setting frequently affect intake. Items on the trays seem unappealing or too difficult to swallow. Food preparation often lacks personal care and service schedules are irregular, especially for those on modified regimens. Breakfast, generally the best meal for hospitalized patients, often is missed because tests and blood drawings must be done while patients are fasting. Patients are taken from their wards for procedures and treatment during morning and early afternoon hours. Once they return to the room, they are visited by doctors, nurses, consultants, and other technical personnel. By the time dinner comes, they are tired, hassled, and lacking whatever appetite they may have had earlier. Thus the frequency of missed meals contributes to the problem of weight loss and poor intake.

Many times a more conducive atmosphere and foods from home or outside sources encourage better intake. For example, if family members can be present during mealtime or if patients are able to eat away from their bed, they frequently have more desire and more willingness to eat. Approval from the attending physician and the dietitian of specially brought in foods must be secured so that the health care team is aware of the types and amounts of these items. Contraindications and restrictions must of course take precedence.

When therapeutic diets are prescribed, it is critical that the nursing staff be aware of patient compliance. This may entail compliance with restrictions. Foods that are not allowed should not be consumed. Just as important is the knowledge that the patient is actually eating the foods provided. If the current modality is not meeting the patient's needs, intervention should occur by advancing to an alternative method of feeding.

If physical limitation is a problem, recommendations for a standby assistant or volunteer during meals should be requested. If depression or emotional reactions seem to be interfering with intake, psychiatric consultation may be appropriate. One method of solving the problem of loneliness or eating alone is to allow the patient to eat elsewhere than in bed.

When patients are required to have between-meal snacks or supplements kept at bedside, adequate cooling and convenient equipment should be supplied such as straws, cups, and special utensils. Compliance with between-meal feedings should be stressed both to the professional staff and the patients. Encouraging patients to complete the required volume or amount of food is important. This takes support from the professional staff and family and also demands some personal motivation on the part of the patients.

Some formulas may be poorly tolerated by mouth. Products vary in consistency and taste. Therefore a mini taste test of several products varying in viscosity, flavor, and caloric density can be offered to determine the patient's preference. Sometimes altering flavor, density, or temperature will aid in compliance.

With this type of feeding, it is important that the nursing staff be aware of formula or contents being spilled out, poured into a cup, and then not used, or not being taken for other reasons. If the patient is not complying with the orders to consume the volume that has been designated, adequate intake will not be achieved and the patient's nutritional status will decline.

ALTERNATIVES TO ORAL INTAKE

At times patients are incapable of meeting their nutritional needs orally, or have contraindications for oral ingestion such as total inability to swallow, obstruction, or surgical procedures. In such instances, tube feeding is an excellent alternative if the bowel is functioning below the point at which the end of the tube is placed.

Tube feeding is commonly underused but is nutritionally the most efficient and cost-effective method of managing patients who are malnourished. The tube can be one of several types: orogastric, nasopharyngeal, nasogastric, or nasojejunal. For patients who may be on long-term tube feedings or are unable to have a tube passed, esophagostoma, gastrostoma, or jejunostoma tubes may be the most appropriate method of feeding (see Chapter 10). With new small-bore soft Silastic, polyurethane, or silicone tubes now available, tolerance is excellent for patients in whom nasal tube placement is feasible.

By tube feeding, the clinician is assured that the patient receives a specific volume containing a selected amount of protein, calories, fat, vitamins, minerals, and trace elements. Those needing predigested formulas will have to be fed by tube due to the unpalatability of these nutrients. With appropriate tube feeding site and bore size, patients now may receive good quality, high-calorie, nutritionally complete diets in whatever form and volume they require.

A variety of delivery systems and methods of tube feeding is available. Funnels or syringes for bolus feedings still are used, but should be carefully evaluated. Gravity or bolus feedings should each take 20 to 40 minutes. Small, frequent feedings are tolerated best by most patients. Those who lack the tolerance or capacity to handle bolus feedings should be fed by a slow-drip method.

Patients who have serious malabsorption, diarrhea, easy satiety, low bowel fistulas, or partial bowel obstruction should have the feeding given slowly, using a tube diameter that is appropriate for the viscosity of the formula (see Appendix 8.C). The concentration of the formula should be increased gradually from half-strength to full-strength as tolerated. The rate of flow is a major factor in acceptability of most formulas. The patient always should be angulated at 30 degrees or higher during and shortly after feeding to diminish regurgitation. The tube should be flushed with water after each feeding. Several inexpensive, easy to operate enteral feeding pumps are available to assure even and continuous flow rates.

When the patient has tried the various types of gastrointestinal feedings using the tract and these have either proved unsuccessful or are no longer appropriate, parenteral nutrition may be the management of choice (see Chapter 9). Parenteral nutrients can be administered peripherally using isotonic concentrations of glucose, crystalline amino acids, and fats, or centrally through a high-flow vein in which hypertonic glucose, together with crystalline amino acids, fats, electrolytes, vitamins, and trace elements are given. This technique does require special procedures and management of the patient. It should be used only if the patient has an obstructed intestine or a fistula, if bowel rest is required, or if the patient is so debilitated that the gastrointestinal tract is nonfunctional. It is the most expensive method of feeding and should only be used as the final choice in nutritional management after all other possibilities have been exhausted. With the information known about nutrition combined with the sophisticated tools and techniques that are available, no patient should become malnourished or develop any kind of nutritional problem.

Once nutrition therapy is begun, electrolytes must be monitored for appropriate response. If the patient does not respond within a day or two or responds inappropriately, the regimen must be adjusted. Finding the right combination may require several modifications or changes. With proper management, the patient will begin to respond positively. It is essential that there be adequate follow-up after discharge from hospital in an effort to assure that nutritional gains made in the hospital are not lost. Too frequently, posthospital care, whether given in an outpatient clinic or by a private physician, does not consider the patient's nutritional status.

Once nutritional requirements are stabilized, discharge planning for home management should begin. If modification of feeding is required, plans should be made to begin training while the patient still is hospitalized.

If the plans include tube feeding, several factors must be considered. Is the patient able to insert the tube and remove it for each feeding? It is not only possible but desirable to have this option available if the medical or surgical condition permits it. A nurse or physician can train a patient in this technique in 10 to 15 minutes. Patients with extensive cortical disease and learning disorders will take longer. The patient then can practice while still in the hospital and be comfortable with the procedure by the time of discharge.

Formula selection depends on the patient's medical, metabolic, and physical needs. If no modifications are required, many foods that the family uses for meals can be adapted for the tube-fed patient using a blender or food processor. When the family's meals are not easily adapted, baby meats, cheese, or cooked eggs can serve as protein sources. Canned or cooked vegetables and canned or ripe fruits may be used. When using foods from the table, the patient may feel more a part of the family and less of a burden; however, care must be taken to ensure that an adequate, well-balanced diet is being consumed (see Appendix 8.D).

If the patient is not physically able to eat or does not have the facilities for using regular food items, a commercially available formula may be the easiest and safest way to provide balanced daily intake. When bowel function is normal, a formula that contains some residue should be selected. Several products consisting of blenderized foodstuffs are available (see Appendix 8.E). Some also come with low-sodium and lactose-free content for patients who need these restrictions, for example, those who are at risk for constipation or fecal impaction.

For patients who are stable and require tube feeding because of physical or mechanical limitations, intermittent bolus feeds are appropriate. The skills needed to self-feed by this method are easily learned. The clinician should note the patient with limited mobility of the upper extremity if hanging a funnel or bag is required. A realistic method will need to be worked out prior to discharge if such a patient is to implement feeding at home.

Patients also can be taught to tube-feed themselves with a pump if slow, continuous feeding is needed. The enteral feeding pumps now available are simple, convenient, and easy to handle. Many patients now are being sent home with this type of equipment and are managing it successfully without assistance. Thorough training in the use of the pump, care of the feeding tube, and maintenance of the equipment should precede discharge. This eliminates mechanical failures that could interfere with nutritional intake.

Patients adapt extremely well to home management and are grateful for having this alternative available. It allows them to be in their familiar home setting and still be able to maintain their nutritional status.

SUMMARY

Nutrition is a major concern to most patients. When weight loss occurs, patients and their families become anxious, distraught, and fearful. Today technology and resources allow patients to be nourished even when they do not have the ability to eat or swallow adequately or effectively. We now can provide various types of nutrition in different forms to meet all patients' needs.

REFERENCES

Allardyce DB, Groves AC. A comparison of nutritional gains resulting from intravenous and enteral feeding. Surg Gynecol Obstet 1974;139:179–84.

Bistrian BR, Blackburn GL, Vitale J, Cochrand D, Naylor J. Prevalence of malnutrition in general medical patients. JAMA 1976;235:1567–70.

Bloch AS. Developing nutrition screening assessment forms. Am J Intra Ther Clin Nutr 1980;746:17–25.

Shils ME. Defined formulas diets for medical purposes. Chicago: American Medical Association, 1977.

Shils ME. Indices of the nutritional status of the individual. In: Selvy N, White PR, eds. Nutrition in the 1980s: constraints on our knowledge. New York: Alan R. Liss, 1981.

Shils ME, Bloch AS, Chernoff R. Liquid formula for oral and tube feeding. New York: Memorial Sloan-Kettering Cancer Center, 1979.

Appendix 8.A

Commercially Available Milk-Based Products to Supplement Intake

C.I.B.

Meritene Liquid

Meritene + Milk

Sustacal + Milk

Sustagen + Water

These products all contain milk and therefore have significant lactose content. They taste the best of all commercial preparations and are among the least expensive. These items will meet the nutritional needs of a patient if given in large enough volumes, but are usually used in smaller volume to augment inadequate intake of solids. Since palatability is high, a great degree of compliance is usually found. Products come in a variety of flavors or can be flavored to taste. Meritene comes in a ready-to-use, pop-top can; the others are powdered and must be reconstituted. Caloric density varies and also depends on accuracy of reconstitution. Products may be purchased in food markets and drugstores without prescription.

Appendix 8.B

Commercially Available Oral or Tube Products For Supplemental or Total Intake

Ensure
Ensure HN
Ensure Plus
Ensure Plus HN
Entrition
Isocal
Isocal HCN
Isotein HN
Magnacal
Nutri-Aid
Osmolite
Osmolite HN
Precision HN
Precision Isotonic
Precision LR
Renu
Travasorb MCT
Travasorb Liquid
Sustacal Liquid HC
Sustacal HC

All products have the following in common:

1.   Contain protein isolates
2.   Contain long-chain carbohydrates
3.   Are lactose free

4.   Are generally palatable
5.   May be taken by mouth or by tube
6.   Are at least 1 calorie per cc caloric density

The following are specific characteristics of individual products:

1.   1.5 calorie per cc—Ensure Plus, Ensure Plus HN, Sustacal HC
     2.0 calorie per cc—Magnacal, Travasorb MCT, Isocal HCN
2.   Unsweetened, unflavored—Entrition, Isocal, Osmolite, Osmolite HN, Isocal HCN
3.   No appreciable fat—Precision LR, Precision HN
4.   Highest protein per 1,000 kcal (24 percent of calories)—Isotein, Sustacal Liquid
5.   Lowest sodium per 1,000 kcal—Isocal HCN, Travasorb MCT
6.   Lowest potassium per 1,000 kcal—Magnacal, Osmolite, Precision LR, Isocal HCN
7.   MCT oil as major fat source—Osmolite, Osmolite HN, Travasorb MCT
8.   Oligosaccharides or malto-dextrins as major carbohydrate source—Entrition, Isocal, Isocal HCN, Isotein HN, Precision HN, Precision Isotonic, Precision LR
9.   Isotonic—Entrition, Isocal, Isotein HN, Osmolite, Osmolite HN, Precision Isotonic, Renu

Appendix 8.C

Defined Formulas for Special Tube Feeding Needs

Criticare HN

Travasorb HN

Travasorb Standard

Vipep

Vital

Vivonex

Vivonex HN

Vivonex TEN

This group of products is designed for those few patients who have compromised digestion, absorption, or use of nutrients. These formulas have hydrolyzed proteins and/or crystalline amino acids for patients who lack the ability to split intact protein efficiently or absorb nutrients readily. Once a protein is split, the palatability of the formula is compromised. Therefore, these products are best administered by tube. All are 1 calorie per cc and are lactose free. All are powdered and must be reconstituted, except Criticare, which comes ready to use. Special characteristics:

1. Greater than 15 percent total kcal as protein—Travasorb HN, Vital, Vivonex HN, Vivonex TEN
2. Medium chain triglyceride oil as major fat source—Travasorb HN, Travasorb Standard, Vipep
3. Low fat—Criticare, Vivonex, Vivonex HN, Vivonex TEN
4. Fat, 10 percent of total kcal—Vital
   Fat, 12 percent of total kcal—Travasorb Standard, Travasorb HN
5. Low sodium—Vital, Vivonex, Vivonex TEN
6. Low potassium—Vivonex TEN
7. Oligosaccharides as carbohydrate source—Travasorb HN, Travasorb Standard, Vivonex, Vivonex HN

Appendix 8.D

Blenderized Tube Feeding Formula

This formula is based on a normal, well-balanced diet. The proportions have been carefully calculated to supply 2,000 calories and adequate protein, minerals, and vitamins.

1 cup enriched farina, cooked

3 eggs, cooked

4 tablespoons skim milk powder

7 ounces ground, lean meat, cooked

1/2 cup carrots, canned

1/2 cup wax beans, canned

1/4 cup corn oil

1½ cups orange juice

1/2 cup dark Karo syrup

1/2 teaspoon salt

2 cups water and juice from canned vegetables

1 multivitamin tablet

Equipment needed:

Blender

Standard measuring cups

Standard measuring spoons

Large household mesh strainer

Mixing bowl or container, 4-quart capacity

Containers to keep formula in refrigerator, such as easily cleaned quart glass bottles or jars (three each)

Bottle brush for washing jars

Method of preparation:

1.   Make fresh daily.
2.   Meat may be lean, ground round of beef or cooked turkey, chicken, or lean cooked beef. If raw beef is used, cook it until it loses its red color. Drain off fat. If cooked meat is used, trim off skin and gristle, cut into cubes.
3.   Cook the farina and eggs. The eggs may be scrambled in some of the oil allowance or stirred into the hot farina.
4.   Always start with some liquid in the blender (about 1 cup).
5.   Add some solid ingredients, a small amount at a time, until the blender is half full.
6.   Blend until smooth.
7.   Pour through the strainer into the large container.
8.   Repeat the small batches until all the ingredients are used.
9.   Vitamin tablet is to be thoroughly crushed with a spoon, added directly to the last batch, and blended for a few minutes.
10. Add water, if necessary, to make a total quantity of 2,000 cc or 2¼ quarts. This will give five feedings of 400 cc (14 oz) per feeding.
11. Store the formula in clean containers in the refrigerator.
12. Warm the formula to room temperature or luke warm by setting the portion in a warm water bath before feeding.

In an emergency, baby foods may be substituted to meet requirements. Carnation Instant Breakfast is also an acceptable emergency substitute if milk products are tolerated well and meet requirements.

Appendix 8.E

Commercially Available Blenderized Products for Tube Feedings

Compleat-B Modified

Compleat-B

Vitaneed

These products are natural blenderized foods that are designed to be used for tube-feeding patients who have head or neck complications or mechanical limitations, not those with specific metabolic or gastrointestinal tract requirements. Compleat-B has a higher sodium content than the other three formulas. Compleat-B Modified and Vitaneed are lactose free for patients who may be lactose intolerant. Although these formulas can be taken by mouth under special circumstances, tube feeding is recommended. All come ready to use in cans, jars, or glass bottles in serving sizes.

CHAPTER 9

Nursing Management of Swallowing Disorders
Barbara A. Griggs

Nurses have the best opportunity to discover a patient who is having difficulty swallowing. Basic knowledge of the anatomy and physiology of normal swallowing aids in alerting nurses to the potential problems and complications of dysphagia. Initial signs and symptoms include a subtle refusal to eat, coughing, choking, drooling, and pain. Awareness of these signs is important, particularly in older, malnourished, or chronically ill patients with no previous history of a swallowing disorder. Other patients of all ages who require careful evaluation of swallowing are those who have recently been transferred from special care units. Prior endotracheal intubation, especially for prolonged periods of time, can contribute to temporary or permanent vocal cord paralysis, leading to difficulty in swallowing and subsequent aspiration (Shapiro, Harrison, and Trout, 1975). It is well established that patients with tracheostoma tubes in place have swallowing difficulties and need careful monitoring for aspiration (Cameron, Reynolds, and Zuidema, 1973; Taylor, Mhoon and Matz, 1981). Nurses should be conscious of these possibilities as a routine part of daily patient assessment. Patients with documented mechanical or neurogenic swallowing disorders need specialized care plans with specific therapeutic goals. Proper hydration, patent airways and nutritional support are requisite areas of meticulous and comprehensive nursing care. This chapter addresses each area with emphasis on providing timely and safe nutritional support.

HYDRATION

Thirst is the physiologic mechanism that governs hydration under normal circumstances. It is important to distinguish between thirst that can be sensed by patients who can take nothing by mouth and intubated or dysphagic patients, and that caused by failure to provide sufficient intravenous or oral fluids.

The initial and most common method of hydration in these patients is intravenous administration of physiologic solutions of water, dextrose, sodium, and potassium chloride. These solutions are administered through a needle or catheter inserted into a peripheral vein. The site of needle or catheter insertion should be changed every two to three days, or more frequently if necessary (Goldmann et al., 1973). Care of the infusion site includes hourly inspection for infiltration, pain, inflammation, or infection. Application of a povidone-iodine ointment and change of dry, sterile dressing once a day is generally accepted practice. Solutions are prepared on the patient care unit or under laminar flow hoods in the pharmacy every 24 hours. Administration set tubing, however, may be changed on a 24- or 48-hour basis according to hospital policy (Buxton et al., 1979). The unit nurse hangs the solution and monitors the infusion carefully, recording the rate and volume infused on a flow chart kept at the bedside. Hourly monitoring is necessary to ascertain complete delivery of required solutions and prevent fluid overload. Twenty-four-hour intake and output totals are also recorded as part of the patient's permanent record. Most routine intravenous solutions are administered by gravity drip. An infusion-control device may be used when solution volumes are restricted.

In addition to basic fluid and electrolyte balance, parenteral solutions may be needed to administer medications. The patient may not be able to swallow the medication or, in the case of certain antibiotics, intravenous infusion may be the preferred route. Many medications are irritating to the vein wall, and therefore proper dilution and frequent site monitoring are essential to prevent phlebitis and potentially serious infiltrations.

MAINTAINING CLEAR AIRWAYS

Management of secretions is one of the first concerns encountered by patients who are having difficulty swallowing. This problem may have causes unrelated to dysphagia (i.e., dental work, fractures, oral tumors, etc.). It is important to distinguish between oral incompetence (such as drooling) and dysphagia that leads to pooling of secretions in the pharynx. Some patients with obstructive tumors or strictures of the esophagus may respond to surgical or irradiation therapy with relief of the anatomic problem. Swallowing retraining may be possible for those with neurologic disorders (see Chapters 5 and 6). Patients require extra care during the time that they are unable to handle their own secretions. Ambulatory and alert patients take care of their immediate needs when provided with proper receptacles and tissues. Bedridden or partially paralyzed patients require more assistance, including a properly supplied bedside stand that is within reach, and an aware nursing staff to respond promptly to their individual needs. Frequent short visits to check on the patient and change receptacles should be routine. The patient should be kept lying on one side and be turned every two hours. A protective pad or soft towel arranged over the pillow under the patient's head will collect saliva from drooling. This should be changed as often as necessary and accompanied by routine skin care to prevent unnecessary chapping. A dental suction tip with gentle suction to remove secretions may be helpful for many patients. The tip must be properly supported and repositioned every hour to prevent pressure points and possible skin breakdown. Alert patients can be taught to use this device by themselves.

Patients with tracheostoma tubes in place require special respiratory care. Many hospitals have chest physical therapists working with such patients on a daily basis. Staff nurses, however, must be trained in tracheostoma care, including proper suctioning technique (Table 9.1).

Adequate ventilation is the first consideration for patients with a tracheostomy tube whether or not they are using a respirator. Routine suctioning every hour and as necessary prevents mucus build-up, tracheal obstruction, and hypoxemia. Aseptic technique is the second consideration, and cannot be overemphasized. Contamination of suction catheters and other related equipment can lead to pneumonia and compromised respiratory function (Shapiro et al., 1975; Egan, 1977; Causey, 1981). Third is avoidance of trauma to the mucous membranes of the trachea by proper suctioning (Nielsen, 1980). Providing adequate nutritional support is often overlooked or is initiated too late. Nutritional repletion and maintenance are essential to prevent breakdown of respiratory musculature and progressive inability of the patient to breathe independently (Doekel et al., 1976; Waxman and Shoemaker, 1980). Finally, patient education and communication are vital. Patients who are unable to talk or call for help become anxious, which may contribute to a decrease in their ventilatory capacity. Continuous explanations of what is happening and why will help to allay their fears. A clipboard with paper and pencil and a bell or buzzer give them a way to communicate. Patients in special care areas become dependent upon the constant presence of nursing staff. Therefore, sufficient preparation must precede the transfer to a regular care unit. A private duty nurse for several days and particularly at night may ease this transition. For some patients, regular visitation by individual family members may be enough.

A major complication of tracheostomy is the development of a tracheoesophageal (TE) fistula. This can be caused by an overinflated cuff creating a pressure point with subsequent erosion (Hedden, Ersoz, and Safar, 1969; Cooper and Grillo, 1977). Proper inflation and the use of double-cuffed tracheostoma tubes or low-pressure cuffs help to minimize this possibility. Coincident use of nasogastric tubes for suction or feeding increase liability to a TE fistula. Large, 16 to 18 French polyvinylchloride nasogastric tubes should be used only for gastric suctioning; it is no longer necessary or recommended to use them for feeding. The availability of small, soft nasogastric feeding tubes has markedly decreased the risk of TE fistula (Figure 9.1).

The most frequent complication of nasogastric feedings is aspiration of food or gastric contents. It is important to note that an inflated tracheostoma (or endotracheal) tube cuff is not a guarantee against this. Signs and symp-

Table 9.1.   How to Suction a Tracheostoma.

Procedure	Rationale
Prepare patient.	Less traumatic for the patient.
Wash hands.	Prevents spread of nosocomial organisms.
Put on sterile glove.	Only the hand holding the suction catheter needs to be gloved.
Attach catheter to wall outlet.	
Lubricate catheter tip with sterile saline solution.	Aids catheter insertion.
Remove ventilator or humidifier apparatus.	
Oxygenate patient with several deep breaths.	Prevents hypoxemia.
Insert catheter quickly but evenly into the trachea WITHOUT suction.	Prevents trauma to mucous membranes.
Start to remove catheter before applying suction.	
Gently roll catheter while smoothly withdrawing it.	
Reoxygenate patient and observe.	
Rinse catheter and connecting tubing with saline noting nature of secretions.	Changes of consistency, color, or odor should be documented.
Repeat procedure once if necessary.	Do not suction patient excessively at one time to prevent bronchospasms and hypoxemia.
Suction oropharyngeal cavity.	This is done after tracheal suctioning to prevent contamination (if necessary to do first, a new catheter and glove are required).
Discard catheter, glove, and saline solution.	Prevents contamination, primarily with *Pseudomonas*.
Reorganize suction materials to be available at all times.	

toms of aspiration include increased respiratory rate with labored breathing, pulmonary congestion with decreased breath sounds, cyanosis, and sweating (diaphoresis). These patients may also manifest a persistent low-grade fever. Those who are dependent on a ventilator should not be fed into the stomach

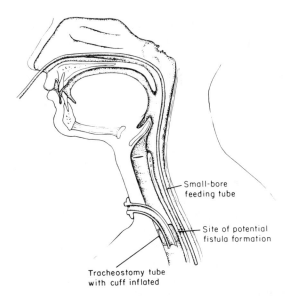

Small-bore
feeding tube

Site of potential
fistula formation

Tracheostomy tube
with cuff inflated

Figure 9.1.   Site of potential tracheoesophageal
fistula.

because the chances of aspiration are much greater. Nasojejunal or intravenous feedings are preferred. It is probably best to wait until a patient has
been weaned from the respirator before beginning nasogastric or oral feedings.

Guidelines for oral feeding of a patient with a tracheostoma are essentially the same as those described for the patient with a swallowing disorder
in the following section. Exceptions include:

1.   The tracheostoma cuff is moderately inflated prior to and for one hour
following the feeding. (Patients may learn to swallow without aspiration
and no longer require a cuffed tube.)
2.   A test for aspiration consists of adding food coloring to a soft food
such as applesauce. The tube is suctioned before the test and the patient
is allowed to rest, then fed two teaspoons of the colored food. After
15 minutes, the tube is gently suctioned just beyond the end. The
returns will be streaked with color if the patient has aspirated; in this
circumstance feedings should be discontinued and the patient reeval-
uated.

NUTRITIONAL SUPPORT

Nosocomial starvation and malnutrition incident to studies and therapy have
been reported in up to 50 percent of hospitalized patients (Bistrian et al.,

1974, 1977). Care givers must be aware of the rapid rate of development with which hospital-acquired malnutrition may evolve, and then do something about it by learning the current options that exist and incorporating them into daily patient therapy (see Chapter 8, Figure 8.1 and related discussion).

Selected patients who are severely depleted, markedly catabolic, or who exhibit gastrointestinal symptoms require a more extensive evaluation, which is frequently done by a member of a specialized nutritional support service where available (Grant, 1980). Anthropometric measurements, nitrogen balance studies, recall antigen skin testing, and oxygen consumption studies are some of the more advanced methods of nutritional assessment (Long et al., 1979; Blackburn et al., 1977). The cumulative results are then used to establish an appropriate feeding method and schedule. It is important to note that the evaluation of nutritional status is an ongoing process that requires reassessment as the patient's clinical condition changes.

There are two primary feeding options: enteral, using the gastrointestinal route, and parenteral, using the intravenous route. The development of parenteral hyperalimentation by Dudrick and colleagues in the late 1960s finally provided the means of feeding patients with nonfunctioning gastrointestinal tracts. Concurrently, elemental diets of simple protein and calorie sources that require minimal digestive capacity provided an alternate method of using the gastrointestinal tract in selected patients (Winitz, Graff, and Gallagher, 1965). This heralded the beginning of specialized nutritional support as we know it today.

While parenteral hyperalimentation is an important medical advancement, patients with swallowing disorders usually have an intact gastrointestinal tract and the goal is to use this first. With special training, some patients may be able to return to oral feedings. For those unable to do so, there still remain two means of access to the gastrointestinal tract through noninvasive and invasive techniques: nasogastric and nasojejunal feeding tubes; and gastrostoma, jejunostoma, and esophagostoma feeding tubes, respectively.

FEEDINGS BY MOUTH

The oral route is the ideal way to provide required nutrients. Oral feeding is not always possible in patients with swallowing disorders, although some can be rehabilitated or trained to this method. The patient's nutritional status and the potential risk of aspiration affect the choice of feeding method. Prior to the availability of parenteral hyperalimentation, there was an urgency to have patients use the gastrointestinal tract as soon as possible, especially those who were depleted. Total parenteral nutrition may make a significant difference in the early rehabilitation of those with dysphagia, but enteral feeding remains the ultimate goal.

A formal evaluation should always precede the decision to initiate oral feedings. Once approved, the nurse's role includes proper patient preparation and supervision.

Positioning

Correct anatomic alignment will help passage of food through pharynx and esophagus with less difficulty in breathing and compromise of swallowing. Patients who can be out of bed are supported in a chair with their head and trunk flexed slightly forward. Those who remain in bed will need the head of the bed elevated and a supporting pillow at the lower back. A patient who has difficulty maintaining one position may need additional pillows on either side. A patient who slides may be stabilized by elevating the midsection of the bed or placing a pillow under the knees. A standing position is ideal for patients on circular electric beds. All patients must be relaxed and well supported in order to eat properly.

Mouth Care

Prior to the introduction of food, mouth care serves to moisten the mucous membranes of the oral cavity and stimulate salivation to prevent food sticking and possible choking. It is equally important to assist with mouth care following a meal to be sure that the oral cavity is free of small food particles that could subsequently be aspirated (Silverman and Elfant, 1979).

Suction Equipment

Suction equipment should be kept on standby for patients with a history of swallowing difficulty. It must always be available and functioning properly in case of emergency. It is best, however, to use it only when necessary because suctioning can contribute to gagging with possible regurgitation and aspiration. Patients with permanent tracheostomas requiring routine suctioning need an organized schedule with sufficient rest time before eating to minimize this possibility.

Choice of Foods

One key to successful feeding is the choice of foods. Water is the easiest to take but the hardest to control. It goes down too fast and there is no bulk to stimulate salivation or the action of oral muscles. A semisoft solid is usually better tolerated (Hargrove, 1980). (See Chapters 5 through 7 for the role of food types and their consistency.)

Close Visual Monitoring

The patient should not be left alone at mealtime. A nurse or occupational therapist should be present to assist and observe until the patient is able to swallow satisfactorily. Later the presence of an aide, a family member, or a volunteer may be sufficient. If not in direct attendance, nurses should be alert to potential problems and be prepared to respond quickly if called. Eating takes time and rushing a meal can be hazardous for any patient, but especially for the one with dysphagia, who may also become exhausted by the technical difficulties associated with eating. Smaller, more frequent meals may be better tolerated.

Education

Education of patient and family is a well-established nursing role. Careful explanations of what the nurse is doing and why relieve anxiety and fear and elicit greater cooperation and success. An explanation comes first, but time and patience must follow.

NONINVASIVE TUBE FEEDING METHODS

When a patient is unable to eat by mouth but has a functioning gastrointestinal tract, the best option is tube feeding. Nasogastric feeding tubes and blenderized formulas have been in existence for many years. (See Chapters 7 and 8 for discussions and illustrations of nasogastric tubes and enteral formulas.)

The decision to use a nasogastric or a nasojejunal feeding tube is, in part, based upon the presence or absence of a gag reflex and the risk of aspiration. Patients with some reflex, who are awake and alert, can be fed nasogastrically. For those with absent gag reflexes and a history or incidence of aspiration, the safest method is nasojejunally (Rombeau and Barot, 1981). The difference between these tubes is primarily the size of the weighted tip and the length of tube that is inserted. Nasogastric tubes have small mercury or tungsten weights that are the same diameter as the rest of the tube. Nasojejunal tubes usually have larger bolus weights, also of mercury or tungsten, at their tips to help with their spontaneous passage through the pylorus into the small intestine. The insertion procedure is approximately the same for both. This is outlined step by step in Table 9.2 and Figures 9.2 and 9.3. Modifications for a nasojejunal tube insertion are given in Table 9.3.

Administration

There are two methods of tube feeding, continuous or intermittent. The continuous method is necessary for jejunal feedings or when the patient can

Table 9.2.   Insertion Procedure for Nasogastric Feeding Tube (with guide).

Procedure	Rationale
1. Position patient in bed at a 45 degree angle with a pillow behind the shoulders.	Patients seem more secure in bed than in a chair. Bed height can be adjusted to make insertion easier.
2. Have patient blow nose, and check each nostril for the side that allows for greater air passage.	Nose spray may be helpful for some patients.
3. Place protective drape over patient's chest, and emesis basin and tissues in patient's lap.	The patient and bed area should be kept clean. Difficulties are not expected but they can arise.
4. Ask patient to hold cup of water with the straw.	
5. Lubricate distal end of feeding tube.	Creates less friction and discomfort in nasal passage.
6. Ask patient to tilt head back slightly.	It is easier to insert tube in this position.
7. Insert tip of tube approximately 2 inches into the nostril.	See Figure 9.2.
8. Ask patient to move head back to a normal position.	
9. Advance tube until patient starts to cough, then ask patient to drink water through the straw.	(Figures 9.3 and 9.4). Vagal stimulation causes a reflex cough. Swallowing will close epiglottis to allow passage of tube into esophagus rather than trachea.
10. If there is resistance, ask patient to extend slightly and turn head to one side.	This aids in passing the tube beyond the nasopharynx.
11. If the patient continually coughs or becomes cyanotic, remove tube immediately.	Tube has probably entered the trachea.
12. When patient is quiet, try again, following steps 5 through 9.	
13. Continue advancing tube while patient swallows water until the mark is reached and feeding tube is in the body of the stomach.	(Figure 9.5). Tube should go in by gravity but swallowing makes procedure easier for the patient. Water seems to work better than ice chips for most patients. Rubbing the throat of an unconscious patient helps to stimulate swallowing. The tube should always be measured for the individual patient to help ensure proper tip location.
14. Loop exposed end of feeding tube, hold securely with left hand approximately 3 inches from the nostril, and gently but firmly pull out plastic guide with right hand.	(Figure 9.6). Patient may feel more comfortable holding tube to keep it from partially pulling out.

Table 9.2. *(continued)*

Procedure	Rationale
15. Check position of feeding tube.	Tube position MUST be checked before feeding begins.
Gently aspirate stomach contents with 50-ml syringe.	An adapter may be needed for a more secure seal. Tubes smaller than 8 French have a tendency to collapse on themselves and therefore should be used primarily when aspiration is not a factor or for supplemental feedings (this refers to nasogastric tubes).
With a stethoscope over left upper quadrant, instill 10 ml of air into feeding tube with syringe.	The sound of air entering stomach can be heard. With smaller tubes, 20 ml of air may be necessary.
Obtain an x-ray if there is any question of tube position	Tubes are radiopaque to enable visualization.
16. Tape feeding tube in place.	Tube must be secure to prevent accidental slippage.
Cleanse nose and cheek with alcohol wipe.	To remove perspiration and skin oils.
Pour tincture of benzoin onto sponge and wipe nose, cheek, and tube. Let air dry.	To protect skin and aid with adherence of tape.
Apply small piece of adhesive tape, with one split end to nose. Wrap ends in opposite directions around the tube.	Adhesive tape seems to adhere best. Too large a piece can focus patient's attention to tip of his nose. When it is necessary to avoid tape, cotton tracheostomy tape can be tied around tube and then around patient's head. Avoid pressure on nostril to prevent subsequent breakdown.
Use tape to secure tube to cheek.	(Figure 9.7). Alert, cooperative patients can use only cheek tape to secure feeding tube. Change tape as necessary.
Loop tubing over ear and plug end of tube.	To prevent tension and air entering tube.

   This is the procedure with a conscious, cooperative patient. An assistant may be necessary if patient is unconscious or uncooperative.

tolerate only small volumes of formula. For some patients, continuous feedings are better absorbed, thus increasing the number of calories provided on a daily basis. Intermittent feedings are given hourly or every three to four hours. They are generally initiated on an hourly basis, and graduated in schedule toward less frequent, larger-volume feedings. This becomes es-

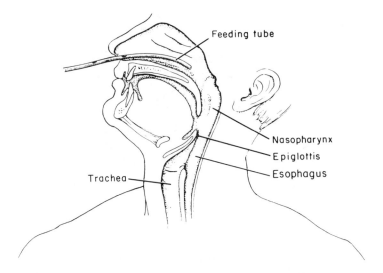

Figure 9.2.   Insertion of feeding tube into the nostril.

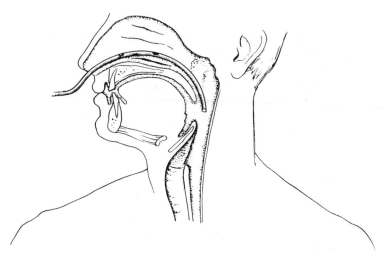

Figure 9.3.   The feeding tube is guided into the nasopharynx.

pecially important if the patient will be continuing tube feedings on hospital discharge.

Tube feedings have been routinely administered by gravity drip; however, with the development of enteral hyperalimentation, enteral feeding pumps have been frequently used. These pumps are less complicated than intravenous infusion devices and also less expensive (Figure 9.9). They enable more accurate administration of continuous feedings and save nursing time, although their purchase is an economic decision made by the hospital.

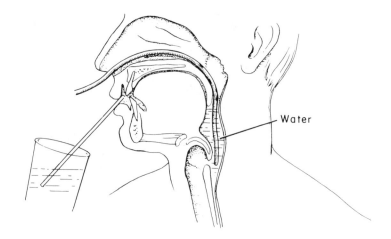

Figure 9.4.   Advancement of the feeding tube with the water bolus.

Whether tube feedings are administered continuously or intermittently, by gravity drip or by feeding pump, they all should start slowly with small volumes. The amount is then increased every day, as tolerated, until the patient's caloric requirement has been met. This may take five to ten days depending on formula osmolarity and patient tolerance. When the maintenance rate has been achieved, adjustments can be made in the frequency and total volume of each feeding. The average adult 70-kg male, nonstressed patient will need 30 to 35 kcal per kg, or a range of 2,100 to 2,400 calories per day. Surgery and sepsis increase patient requirements to 40 to 45 kcal per kg (Walters and Freeman, 1981).

Complications

The two main complications associated with tube feedings are aspiration and diarrhea. Decreased incidence or prevention of both can be accomplished by adhering to the following guidelines:

1.   Elevate the head of the bed at least 30 degrees during feeding and for one hour after feeding.
2.   Aspirate the feeding tube every two hours to check for absorption of the formula. Progressively increasing residual volumes, nausea, abdominal distention, and discomfort should alert the nurse to hold the feeding and notify the physician to re-evaluate the patient. Residual volumes of 150 to 200 ml should be questioned.
3.   Administer intermittent feedings by slow, gravity drip rather than as a bolus.

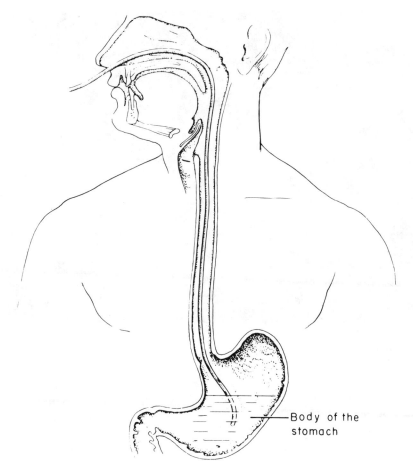

Body of the
stomach

Figure 9.5.   Correct positioning of the feeding tube in the stomach.

4.   Coordinate with the dietitian the most appropriate formula for the patient.
5.   Administer antidiarrheal preparations as necessary.
6.   Monitor fluid and electrolyte balance daily.

INVASIVE FEEDING METHODS

Patients who require tube feedings for prolonged or indefinite periods of time should be considered candidates for a gastrostomy, jejunostomy, or esophagostomy. Surgical insertion of feeding tubes into the stomach, intestine, or esophagus is a sterile procedure that may necessitate general anesthesia. It may be a relatively short, minor procedure or a more extensive,

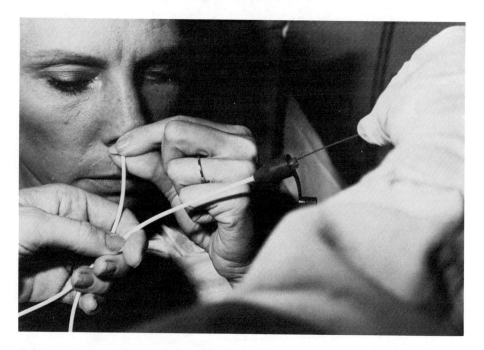

Figure 9.6.   Removal of the monofilament guide from the feeding tube.

major one depending upon the choice of procedure and the patient's condition. Occasionally, procedures are performed under local anesthesia in selected patients when general anesthesia is risky or contraindicated. Development of the needle-catheter jejunostomy has increased the use of this access route (Delaney, 1973; Delaney et al., 1977). (For a detailed explanation of these surgical procedures see Chapter 10.)

The nursing care of a patient with an ostomy tube includes keeping the tube intact and patent, preventing local skin irritation, providing accurate infusions, and monitoring for potential complications.

Procedure for keeping the tube intact and patent depends on the type of tube that is inserted. All tubes are sutured in place at least initially, but inadvertent tension primarily from the administration tubing and connector can contribute to its dislodgment. Many tubes used for gastrostomies are large, 16 to 18 French, and therefore need to be taped more securely. Adhesive tape remains one of the best to do this. The tape should be pinched completely around the tube, leaving about one to one and a half inches of tape on either side for adherence. Jejunostoma tubes are smaller, 5 to 8 French, but longer. The additional tubing should be coiled and taped securely, with a protective gauze covering, until the site is healed and when not in use. Esophagostoma tubes vary from red rubber catheters to smaller, soft, weighted tubes. The tubes may be sutured until a tract is formed. For

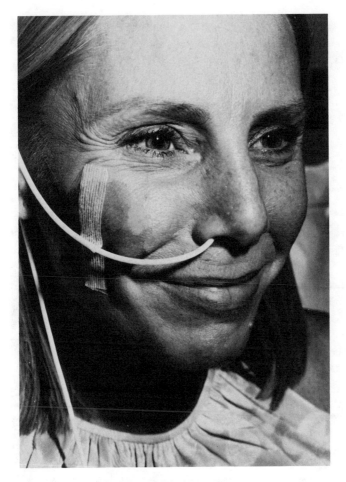

Figure 9.7.   Steri-strip taping of the feeding tube.

Table 9.3.   Modifications for Insertion of Nasojejunal Feeding Tube.

Insert an additional 25 to 35 cm of tubing into stomach.
Wait for tube passage into intestines:
   1 to 2 hours for ambulatory patients.
   24 hours or more for bedridden patients.
   If tube does not pass spontaneously, manual passage by endoscopy may be necessary.
Document exact position of feeding tube prior to initiation of tube feeding (Figure 9.8).

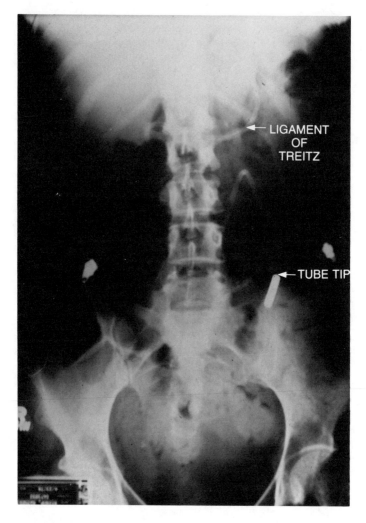

Figure 9.8.   Radiographic documentation of the tip of the nasojejunal feeding tube in the midjejunum must take place before feedings begin.

some patients, the tube can be removed and be reinserted for each feeding. Unlike the noninvasive feeding tubes, gastrostoma/jejunostoma or new esophagostoma feeding tubes require surgical replacement if accidentally pulled out.

Skin cleansing and the application of a skin adherent, such as tincture of benzoin, help to prevent tissue breakdown. Changing the tape as necessary and moving the tube to alternate sides will also help to maintain skin integrity. The ostomy tube exit site is protected by a dry, sterile dressing. When gastrostoma tubes are used, the end of the tube must be clamped and covered with a gauze sponge between feedings to prevent backflow of gastric contents,

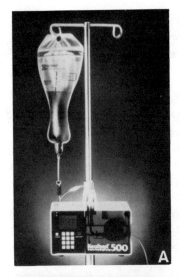
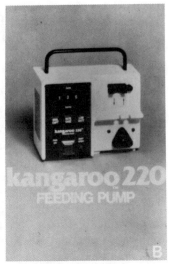
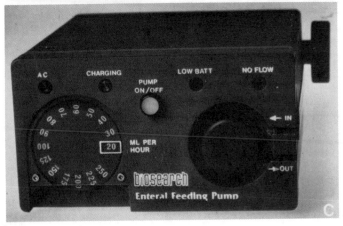

Figure 9.9. Examples of infusion-control devices specific for enteral formulations. (A) Keofeed 500 enteric feeding pump (Keofeed is a registered trademark of IVAC Corporation), (B) Kangaroo 220 feeding pump (courtesy of Chesebrough-Ponds, Inc.), (C) Biosearch enteral feeding pump (courtesy of Biosearch Medical Products, Inc.).

which are extremely irritating. The area around esophagostoma tubes requires more frequent skin care because of the possibility of saliva draining through the opening.

The administration of ostomy tube feedings is essentially the same as for noninvasive tube feedings, with two exceptions. First, patients with esophagostomies rarely have difficulty tolerating larger volumes of formula (350 to 500 ml) administered by gravity drip every three to four hours. We should always be aware, however, that the patients can aspirate. Second, needle-catheter jejunostomies with a 16-gauge catheter require an elemental diet and an infusion control device to guarantee consistent flow (Freeman, Egan, and Millis, 1976).

The complications for ostomy tube feedings include postoperative edema, bleeding, tube dislodgment, and peritonitis as well as aspiration and diarrhea. The surgical procedure is short and nontraumatic for most patients. However, any incision and tissue manipulation can result in edema and bleeding. Small pressure dressings are applied in the operating room and remain in place at least overnight. Proper taping to secure the feeding tube has been previously stressed. Dislodgment could lead to leakage of gastrointestinal secretions into the peritoneal cavity and the possibility of peritonitis (Torosian and Rombeau, 1980). Patients with esophagostomas must also be closely monitored for tracheal obstruction in the early postoperative period.

PARENTERAL NUTRITIONAL SUPPORT

The original indication for total parenteral nutrition (TPN) was for the patient with a nonfunctioning gastrointestinal tract. There are additional indications when adequate oral intake is inappropriate or even hazardous. These include patients who are malnourished or severely depleted and those who have obstructions or inflammation of the central nervous system or upper gastrointestinal tract. For example, a patient who has had a recent cerebrovascular accident and has no protective reflexes is at risk of aspiration. Similarly, a patient receiving irradiation therapy to the oral cavity or esophagus who cannot swallow. These patients can benefit from parenteral nutritional support until their conditions stabilize and a long-range nutritional plan is made. There are two methods of providing parenteral hyperalimentation: central, or total parenteral nutrition (TPN), and peripheral parenteral nutrition (PPN).

Total Parenteral Nutrition

Total parenteral nutrition is the administration of a complete metabolic diet through a central venous route. The components are carbohydrates as hypertonic dextrose, protein as synthetic amino acids, plus essential electrolytes, trace minerals, and vitamins (Dudrick et al., 1969; Shils, 1972). Fat as either soybean or safflower oil is provided separately (Hansen, Hardie, and Hidalgo, 1976; Pelham, 1981). A typical TPN dextrose/amino acid solution contains approximately 25 percent dextrose and 50 gm amino acids in one liter and is equivalent to 1 calorie per ml. The average patient receives 1,800 to 3,000 ml per day. When used as a caloric source, fat comprises one-third of the daily required calories (Meguid et al., 1982). Five hundred milliliters of fat, however, is more likely given only twice a week to prevent essential fatty acid deficiency (Riella et al., 1975; Faulkner and Flint, 1977).

Hypertonic solution is irritating to peripheral veins and for this reason central venous access is necessary. A subclavian or internal jugular vein is used as an entry point for the catheter. This is a sterile procedure performed at the bedside for most patients. The catheter is threaded to its correct position in the superior vena cava; its position is documented by x-ray. The solution is ordered by the physician and prepared daily in the pharmacy under a laminar flow hood. The nurse administers the solution by an infusion-control device to ensure accuracy. In addition, the patient is closely monitored through vital signs, weight, intake and output record, urine spot tests, and routine blood tests of electrolytes, glucose, renal and liver function plus selected other values based on the individual's condition.

The complications of TPN therapy can be significant, and require awareness and professional skill to minimize or prevent their occurrence. Pneumothorax is the most common major complication associated with central venous catheterization (Mitchell and Clark, 1979). Proper patient preparation and physician training will markedly decrease this possibility. The TPN catheter provides direct access to the central bloodstream and the average length of therapy for most acutely ill patients is two to four weeks. Therefore meticulous catheter care is essential. Catheter dressings are changed at least three times a week based on hospital policy and the type of dressing material that is used. The dressing change is a sterile procedure requiring mask and gloves. A defatting agent may be used initially, then a form of povidone-iodine (solution and/or ointment) is applied (Figure 9.10). Small gauze dressings are sufficient to protect the catheter exit site because there is no drainage (Figure 9.11). A skin adhesive is recommended and finally the area is occlusively taped by one of the many tapes currently available (Figure 9.12).

The tubing used to administer TPN solution, including cassettes when used, is changed every 24 hours (Goldmann and Maki, 1973). This can become a routine procedure with the first bottle of each day. Care in handling the solution and tubing is necessary to prevent contamination and possible infection. Proper taping of the tubing will prevent separation at the catheter hub and leakage of solution, blood, or air. A wet dressing increases the chance of infection. Blood back-up can cause the catheter to clot and abrupt cessation of the solution flow, leading to a hypoglycemic episode and catheter replacement. Finally, air leakage may mean an air embolism. All three of these potential complications are avoidable through proper attention to details of care.

The most common metabolic complication of TPN is hyperglycemia because of the high concentrations of dextrose that are infused. To prevent this, one should first start at a low infusion rate, about 30 to 40 ml per hour, and gradually increase the rate over several days while closely monitoring levels of blood and urine sugar. Second, it is important to be aware of those

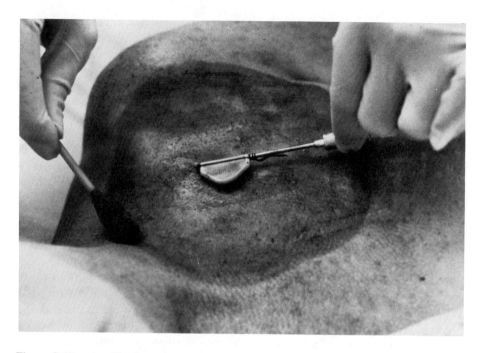

Figure 9.10.   Application of povidone-iodine solution.

patients who are susceptible to glucose intolerance and add regular insulin to the TPN solution as necessary to avoid glucosuria and keep blood glucose levels within normal range (Dudrick et al., 1972). Other metabolic imbalances occur due to the patient's depleted or disease state and can be controlled by additions to or deletions from the TPN solution as determined by regularly scheduled laboratory monitoring. Deficiencies of essential fatty acids and trace minerals were a problem before safe intravenous fat emulsions and trace mineral preparations became available for routine administration.

Peripheral Parenteral Nutrition

Patients who need only short-term parenteral therapy, for example, seven to ten days, before starting oral or tube feedings may be able to benefit from PPN. It is made up of the same components as TPN; however, the dextrose/ amino acid solution is less concentrated and comprises only half of the total therapy volume. The other half is administered as fat. Consequently, it takes one to one and a half liters of dextrose/amino acids and one to one and a half liters of 10 percent fat emulsion to provide approximately 1,400 to 2,000 calories per day (Deitel and Kaminsky, 1974; Freeman, 1978). The advantage of PPN solutions is that they can be administered by peripheral vein. Dis-

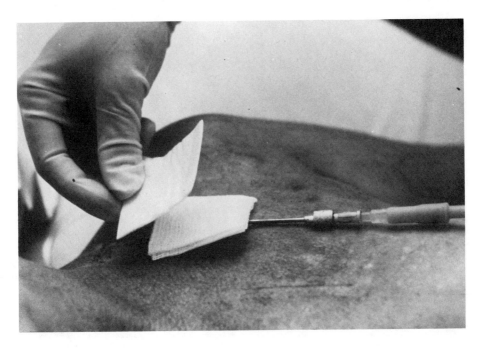

Figure 9.11. Gauze dressings are used to protect the catheter exit site.

advantages are unavailability of peripheral veins and the patient's inability to tolerate the total volume of fluid and fat (Walters and Freeman, 1981). Patients with cardiac or renal disorders, severe liver disease, pulmonary disease, or blood coagulation disorders are rarely candidates for this therapy (Silberman, Freehauf, and Fong, 1977). Unless contraindicated, PPN may be used for the dysphagic patient who is undergoing a feeding trial. This provides sufficient calories without interference of a nasogastric or nasojejunal feeding tube.

A peripheral catheter or needle is inserted under sterile conditions and changed every 48 to 72 hours (Goldmann et al., 1973). The site is inspected hourly for signs of inflammation or infiltration. Solutions are prepared in the pharmacy on a daily basis. They are administered by gravity drip or infusion-control devices, if available, with changes of intravenous tubing every 24 hours. A dry, sterile dressing is changed daily, with similar skin care as with central catheters, although mask and gloves are not worn. Patient monitoring is the same for both TPN and PPN.

Complications of PPN relate mainly to the infusion site. Irritation of the vein wall with painful phlebitis or infiltration is common (Gazitua et al., 1979; Massar et al., 1982). Local infection with bacteremias is rare, but does occur. Too rapid administration may lead to fluid overload and respiratory distress. Each of these complications is preventable with careful and frequent patient observations.

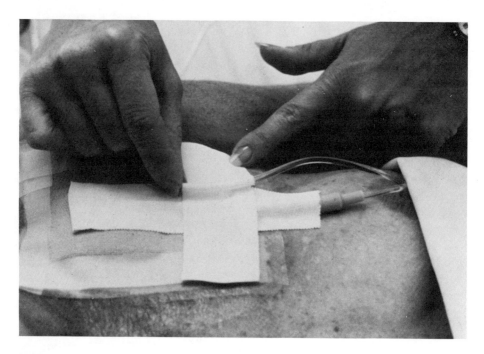

Figure 9.12.   The final occlusive dressing.

SUMMARY

It is important for a nurse to be familiar with the pathology of swallowing disorders, including the differences between those of neurologic, mechanical, and psychiatric origin. The specific signs and symptoms and the current treatment modalities affect daily and long-term care plans for each patient. The nursing management of dysphagic patients requires knowledge, skill, and patience. Attention to proper hydration and clear airways should be followed by early nutritional intervention. There is no question today that nutritional support should be a consideration for each patient. Enteral and parenteral feeding methods are available and provide options, through one or a combination of therapies, to meet the needs of all of our patients.

REFERENCES

Bistrian B, Blackburn G, Hallowell E, Heddle M. Protein status of general surgical patients. JAMA 1974;230:858–60.

Bistrian B, Blackburn G, Vitale J, Cochran D, Naylor J. Prevalence of malnutrition in general medical patients. JAMA 1976;235:1567–70.

Blackburn G, Bistrian B, Maini B, Schlamm H, Smith M. Nutritional and metabolic assessment of the hospitalized patient. J Parent Ent Nutr 1977;1:11–22.

Buxton A, Highsmith A, Garner J, et al. Contamination of intravenous infusion fluid; effects of changing administration sets. Ann Intern Med 1979;90:764–68.

Cameron J, Reynolds J, Zuidema G. Aspiration in patients with tracheostomies. Surg Gynecol Obstet 1973;136:68–70.

Causey W. Infections complicating mechanical ventilation. In: Rattenborg C, Via-Reque E, eds. Clinical use of mechanical ventilation. Chicago, London: Yearbook Medical Publishers, 1981;26:280–91.

Cooper J, Grillo H. Analysis of problems related to cuffs in intratracheal tubes. In: Rogers R, ed. Respiratory intensive care. Springfield, Ill.: Charles C Thomas, 1977;245–60.

Deitel M, Kaminsky V. Total nutrition by peripheral vein—the lipid system. Can Med Assoc J 1974;111:152–54.

Delaney H, Carnevale N, Garvey J. Jejunostomy by a needle-catheter technique. Surgery 1973;73:786–90.

Delaney H, Carnevale N, Garvey J, Moss C. Postoperative nutritional support using needle-catheter-feeding jejunostomy. Ann Surg 1977;186:165–70.

Doekel R, Zwillich C, Scoggin C, Kryger M, Weil J. Clinical semi-starvation; depression of hypoxic ventilatory response. N Engl J Med 1976;295:358–61.

Dudrick S, Macfadyen B, VanBuren C, Ruberg R, Maynard A. Parenteral hyperalimentation; metabolic problems and solutions. Ann Surg 1972;176:259–62.

Dudrick S, Wilmore D, Vars H, Rhoads J. Long-term total parenteral nutrition with growth development and positive nitrogen balance. Surgery 1968;64:134–42.

Dudrick S, Wilmore D, Vars H, Rhoads J. Can intravenous feeding as the sole means of nutrition support growth in the child and restore weight loss in an adult? Ann Surg 1969;169:974–84.

Egan D. Fundamentals of respiratory therapy. St. Louis: C V Mosby, 1977.

Faulkner W, Flint L. Essential fatty acid deficiency associated with total parenteral nutrition. Surg Gynecol Obstet 1977;144:665–67.

Freeman J. Peripheral parenteral nutrition. Can J Surg 1978;21:489–92.

Freeman J, Egan M, Millis B. The elemental diet. Surg Gynecol Obstet 1976;142:925–32.

Gazitua R, Wilson K, Bistrian B, Blackburn G. Factors determining peripheral vein tolerance to amino acid infusions. Arch Surg 1979;114:897–900.

Goldmann D, Maki D. Infection control in total parenteral nutrition. JAMA 1973;223:1360–64.

Goldmann D, Maki D, Rhame F, Kaiser A, Tenney J, Bennett J. Guidelines for infection control in intravenous therapy. Ann Intern Med 1973;79:848–50.

Grant J. A team approach: handbook of total parenteral nutrition. Philadelphia: W B Saunders, 1980.

Hansen L, Hardie B, Hildalgo J. Fat emulsion for intravenous administration: clinical experience with Intralipid 10%. Ann Surg 1976;184:80–88.

Hargrove R. Feeding the severely dysphagic patient. J Neurosurg Nurs 1980;12:102–7.

Hedden M, Ersoz C, Safar P. Tracheoesophageal fistulas following prolonged artificial ventilation via cuffed tracheostomy tubes. Anesthesiology 1969;31:281–89.

Long C, Schaffel N, Geiger J, Schiller N, Blakemore W. Metabolic response to injury and illness: the establishment of energy and protein needs from indirect calorimetry and nitrogen balance. J Parent Ent Nutr 1979;3:452–56.

Luther W, Sykes T. Textbook of parenteral nutrition. New York: Grune and Stratton, not yet published.

Massar E, Daly J, Copeland E, Johnson D, et al. Peripheral vein complications in patients receiving amino acid/dextrose solutions. J Parent Ent Nutr 1982;7:159–62.

Meguid M, Schimmel E, Johnson W, et al. Reduced metabolic complications in total parenteral nutrition: pilot study using fat to replace one-third of glucose calories. J Parent Ent Nutr 1982;6:304–7.

Mitchell S, Clark R. Complications of central venous catheterization. Am J Roentgenol 1979;133:467–76.

Nielsen L. Potential problems of mechanical ventilation. Am J Nurs 1980;80:2206–13.

Pelham L. Rational use of intravenous fat emulsions. Am J Hosp Pharm 1981;38:198–208.

Riela M, Broviac J, Wells M, Scribner B. Essential fatty acid deficiency in human adults during total parenteral nutrition. Ann Intern Med 1975;83:786–89.

Rombeau J, Barot L. Enteral nutrition therapy. In: Mullen J, Crosby L, Rombeau J, eds. The surgical clinics of North America: symposium on surgical nutrition. Philadelphia: WB Saunders 1981;610–11.

Shapiro S, Harrison R, Trout C. Maintenance of artificial airways of extubation. In: Shapiro S et al., eds. Clinical application of respiratory care. Chicago: Yearbook Medical Publishers, 1975;16:254–9.

Shils M. Guidelines for total parenteral nutrition. JAMA 1972:220:1921–29.

Silberman H, Freehauf M, Fong G, Rosenblatt N. Parenteral nutrition with lipids. JAMA 1977;238:1380–82.

Silverman E, Elfant I. Dysphagia: an evaluation and treatment program for the adult. Am J Occup Ther 1979;33:382–92.

Taylor H, Mhoon E, Matz G. Complications due to tracheostomy and endotracheal tubes. In: Rattenborg C, Via-Reque E, eds. Clinical use of mechanical ventilation. Chicago, London: Yearbook Medical Publishers, 1981;25:273–75.

Torosian M, Rombeau J. Feeding by tube enterostomy. Surg Gynecol Obstet 1980;150:918–27.

Walters J, Freeman J. Parenteral nutrition by peripheral vein. In: Mullen J, Crosby L, Rombeau J, eds. The surgical clinics of North America: symposium on surgical nutrition. Philadelphia: W B Saunders, 1981;593–4.

Waxman K, Shoemaker W. Management of postoperative and posttraumatic respiratory failure in the ICU. In: Bartlett R, ed. The surgical clinics of North America: symposium on respiratory care in surgery. Philadelphia: W B Saunders, 1980;1424–25.

Winitz M, Graff J, Gallagher N. Evaluation of chemical diets as nutrition for man-in-space. Nature 1965;205:741–43.

CHAPTER 10

Surgical Intervention in Dysphagia

Harold C. Pillsbury III and Jeffrey A. Buckwalter

The upper aerodigestive tract is a complex neuromuscular structure with dual functions in respiration and deglutition. Abnormalities in deglutition often affect laryngeal function. From an evolutionary point of view, the larynx is primarily a sphincter to protect the upper airway from life-threatening aspiration (Negus, 1962). Management of disorders that cause dysphagia must emphasize the dual role of the structure involved and if possible, specific treatment maneuvers must preserve the function of both systems. The pathologic state that affects deglutition may be categorized as structural (mechanical), such as tumor or foreign body, and functional (neuropathic), such as cranial nerve paralysis or muscle spasm. This chapter presents a logical order of surgical intervention for the patient suffering with severe dysphagia and aspiration as it relates to functional disorders.

Briefly, the act of swallowing includes three stages (see Chapter 1 for details): oral, pharyngeal, and esophageal. The oral stage is voluntary and provides initiation of the subsequent involuntary stages of swallowing by the propulsion of the food bolus into the oropharynx. Dysfunction of the oral stage is least common, but hypoglossal paralysis resulting in the inability to propel secretions and food into the oropharynx limits the success of surgical intervention for pharyngeal stage dysfunction (Lebo, Kwei, and Norris, 1976). The pharyngeal stage of deglutition is a peristaltic sequence of voluntary and involuntary muscular reflexes facilitating the passage of a bolus into the esophagus while preventing nasal and tracheal aspiration. As the bolus enters the pharynx, the soft palate is elevated and the superior constrictor converges medially, sealing the nasopharynx off from the oral cavity. The larynx is elevated and shielded from the bolus by the epiglottis, base of tongue, and to some extent by the soft palate as it enters the hypopharynx. As the larynx is elevated, the hypopharynx relaxes to receive the bolus. As the bolus fills the hypopharynx the constrictor peristalsis begins propelling the bolus toward the esophagus. Temporary relaxation of the cricopharyngeus muscle allows passage of the bolus into the esophagus, initiating esophageal peristalsis, after which the muscle resumes its resting tone.

Dysfunction of the pharyngeal stage of deglutition may involve laryngeal elevation, glottic closure, constrictor contraction, cricopharyngeal relaxation, or the required temporal coordination between constrictor contraction and cricopharyngeal relaxation. In the pharyngeal stage of deglutition, surgical intervention has been successful in relieving dysphagia and aspiration by cricopharyngeal myotomy, a procedure that is discussed extensively later in this chapter.

The final stage of deglutition is esophageal. Once the bolus has traversed the pharyngoesophageal segment, peristalsis and gravity propel it to the inferior esophageal sphincter at the gastroesophageal junction. As the bolus descends in the esophagus, the inferior sphincter relaxes, allowing free passage into the stomach. Dysfunction of the final stage of deglutition may result from inadequate esophageal peristalsis, inappropriate timing, insufficient degree of relaxation of the lower esophageal sphincter, and/or hypotension of the lower esophageal sphincter resulting in esophageal reflux or inordinate, sustained contraction spasm of any portion of the esophagus.

Disease processes resulting in deglutition dysfunction are listed in Table 10.1 (see also Chapter 2). Disorders causing dysphagia that have been managed successfully by surgical intervention are central nervous system, myopathic, postconservation or laryngeal surgery, or idiopathic in etiology (Ellis, 1971). Surgical intervention in these disorders is initially conservative. Only as the degree of dysphagia and associated aspiration increases, as judged by

Table 10.1.   Etiologic Summary of Deglutition Disorders.

Etiology	Disorder
Central nervous system	Bulbar poliomyelitis
	Cerebrovascular accident
	Trauma
	Parkinson's disease
	Multiple sclerosis
	Amyotrophic lateral sclerosis
Myopathy	Muscular dystrophy (myotonic, oculopharyngeal)
	Myasthenia gravis
	Metabolic (thyrotoxicosis, hypothyroidism)
	Carcinomatosis
	Inflammation (dermatomyositis, polymyositis)
Peripheral disease	Trauma
	Neuritis
	Postsurgical conditions
Idiopathic incoordination	Pharyngoesophageal diverticulum

the patient's physical debilitation and presence of recurrent aspiration pneumonia, is more aggressive intervention indicated.

THE CRICOPHARYNGEUS

A common site for dysfunction resulting in dysphagia is the cricopharyngeus muscle. It has been studied extensively and is generally considered to be the superior esophageal sphincter (Asherson, 1950; Kirchner, 1958; Lund, 1968; Ellis, 1971). Inferior to the oblique fibers of the inferior constrictor muscle, the cricopharyngeus muscle forms a sling around the pharyngoesophageal segment from anterior lateral attachments to the cricoid cartilage. Inferiorly, the cricopharyngeus is continuous in some specimens with the superior circular fibers of the esophagus (Hollinshead, 1968). In addition to this anatomic identification of the superior sphincter, manometric measurements reveal a sphincter approximately 2.5 to 6 cm (average 3 cm) in length and having a resting pressure of 18 to 60 cm (average 40 cm) above atmospheric pressure (English, 1980).

Innervation of the cricopharyngeus in man remains controversial (Figure 10.1). In the dog model, Kirchner (1958) conclusively demonstrated the motor supply to the cricopharyngeus muscle to be a pharyngeal branch of the vagus nerve. In man, it is generally considered to be innervated by the pharyngeal nerve plexus, consisting of contributions from the glossopha-

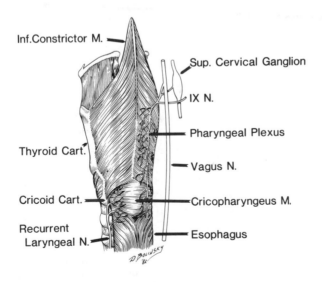

Figure 10.1.   Posterior view of the nerve supply to the cricopharyngeal and pharyngeal musculature. Drawing by David Bolinsky.

ryngeus, vagus, and superior sympathetic ganglion (Blakley, Garety, and Smith, 1968).

The cricopharyngeus muscle, functioning as the superior esophageal sphincter and being the terminal event in the critical pharyngeal stage of deglutition, is identified as contributing significantly to dysphagia. The cricopharyngeus has been studied extensively by manometric measurements; in the pathologic state it may be in spasm (Calcaterra, Kadell, and Ward, 1975; Chodosh, 1975), contract prematurely, be delayed in contraction (Ellis et al., 1969), and contribute significantly to the formation of pharyngoesophageal diverticula (Zenker's diverticulum) (Dohlman and Mattson, 1960; Lund, 1968; Weaver and Fleming, 1978). In some diseases involving deglutition, resistance of a normally functioning superior sphincter is too great for weakened pharyngeal constrictor muscles to overcome, resulting in dysphagia (Blakley, Garety, and Smith, 1968).

Prior to surgical intervention for dysphagia, an extensive evaluation of the upper aerodigestive tract must be completed. The most effective preoperative evaluation includes a cine-esophageal barium swallow, esophagoscopy, and manometric measurements (Orringer, 1980). Often revealed by the barium swallow are a prominent cricopharyngeal sphincter, a prominent posterior cricopharyngeal bar on lateral cervical views, and Zenker's diverticulum (see Figures 4.4 and 4.5). In addition to identifying a functional disorder, intrinsic or extrinsic masses must be eliminated as possible causes of dysphagia.

CRICOPHARYNGEAL MYOTOMY

The most widely practiced management of cricopharyngeal dysfunction has been surgical intervention by performing a cricopharyngeal myotomy (Blakley, Garety, and Smith, 1968; Mills, 1975; Zuckerbraum and Bahma, 1979; Ellis, 1980; Black, 1981) or an extended myotomy (Figure 10.2). Depending on the patient's physical condition, this procedure can be performed under local or general anesthesia. Either an oblique incision anterior to the sternocleidomastoid muscle or a horizontal incision at the level of the cricoid cartilage is made. The left side is preferred by most surgeons. Following sharp dissection through the subcutaneous tissues and the platysma, the larynx is exposed by separating the strap muscles, exposing the cricopharyngeus muscle. The larynx is retracted medially, while the carotid sheath and contents are retracted laterally (Calcaterra, Kadell, and Ward, 1975; Ellis, 1980). The middle thyroid vein often must be cut to facilitate exposure. The recurrent laryngeal nerve must be identified and protected. Critical to the success of the myotomy is identification and division of the cricopharyngeal muscle fibers. One technique to accomplish this goal is to place a bougie (weighted rubber tube) into the esophagus, thus distending the sphincter and allowing all the fibers to be identified and cut, exposing the

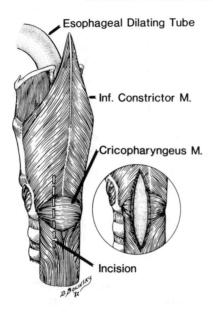

Esophageal Dilating Tube

Inf. Constrictor M.

Cricopharyngeus M.

Incision

Figure 10.2. Incision for the cricopharyngeal myotomy. The inset shows the mucosa bulging through the excised musculature. Drawing by David Bolinsky.

underlying mucosal membrane (Skolnik, Tenta, and Massair, 1966). By this extension, we feel a complete myotomy can be guaranteed. As an additional precaution to prevent recurrent laryngeal nerve injury, the myotomy is performed in the midline on the posterior surface of the esophagus.

Zenker's diverticula are often present in association with cricopharyngeal dysfunction. The base of the diverticulum is located superior to the slinglike band of cricopharyngeus muscle and is inferior to the oblique fibers of the inferior constrictor. Diverticula range in size from small (1 to 3 cm) to large (5 to 8 cm). There is evidence from clinical experience that the size of the diverticulum does not correlate with the degree of dysphagia (Orringer, 1980). This has led to the belief that an adequate myotomy will resolve the symptoms of dysphagia when small diverticula are present. Many surgeons have demonstrated their disappearance by postoperative esophageal swallow in patients having myotomy alone for small diverticula. For large diverticula, surgical resection with two-layer closure of the mucous membrane and myotomy is indicated (Ellis, 1969).

The complications of cricopharyngeal myotomy are few, being primarily incomplete division of the cricopharyngeus muscle resulting in persistent dysphagia, damage to the recurrent laryngeal nerve, and fistula formation from unrecognized perforation of the mucous membrane. Because of these complications and the usual poor systemic condition of the patients, some advocate endoscopic resection of the common wall between the diverticulum and esophagus by coagulating diathermy current (Dohlman and Mattson, 1966). This procedure opens the diverticulum and at the same time divides the cricopharyngeus muscle. The procedure has received only modest acceptance because of limited surgical exposure, a high rate of fistulization, and a lower success rate due to the inability to know when the cricopharyngeus has been completely divided.

Postoperative evaluation of patients having a cricopharyngeal myotomy for dysphagia reveals elimination of dysphagia, or only an occasional episode of mild dysphagia in 85 percent of patients studied (Black, 1981). In addition, manometric measurements demonstrate an approximate 50 percent decrease in the resting pressure of the superior sphincter. Patients who have premature contraction of the sphincter prior to myotomy continue to do so postoperatively (Ellis, 1969), although they have less dysphagia. Patients with multiple cranial nerve dysfunctions, especially the hypoglossal nerve, or those who have significant ballooning of the pharyngeal constrictor muscles preoperatively achieve only a modest improvement in dysphagia after cricopharyngeal myotomy (Lebo, Kwei, and Norris, 1976).

Dilatation of the superior esophageal sphincter using bougie dilators has been advocated as an alternative treatment in patients with idiopathic spasm or achalasia of the superior esophageal sphincter (Calcaterra, Kadell, and Ward, 1975). This treatment is recommended in systemically debilitated patients who cannot tolerate a more involved surgical procedure. Management of superior esophageal achalasia by dilatation is limited in effectiveness because the procedure must be repeated and relief is only short-term. Multiple dilatation of the superior esophagus can result in significant risk of esophageal perforation. Because of the necessity for repeated procedures and the significant morbidity and mortality associated with esophageal perforation, superior esophageal sphincter dilatation for dysphagia is only indicated in a select, small group of patients, such as younger persons who are not debilitated but who demonstrate mild to moderate narrowing. Those who do not respond readily to this treatment should not be considered for long-term repeated dilatation.

Cricopharyngeal myotomy is advocated (Thawley and Ogura, 1978) in patients undergoing conservative surgery of the larynx, including hemilaryngectomy and unilateral and bilateral supraglottic laryngectomy. Following conservative laryngeal surgery for carcinoma and resulting reconstruction, pharyngeal structure and ability to function are altered. Often these patients require weeks to months of practice to relearn the neuromuscular sequence for effective swallowing. By cine-esophageal swallow and manometric pressure measurements, the pharyngeal musculature has been demonstrated to be ineffective in propelling a bolus or secretions through the cricopharyngeal sphincter. A cricopharyngeal myotomy should be considered in these patients and is performed by some surgeons at the time of conservative laryngeal surgery (Nicks, 1976). We perform a myotomy in all patients undergoing supraglottic laryngectomy because there is a tendency for the cricopharyngeus to fail to relax properly following the procedure, and aspiration becomes the significant postoperative problem.

ESOPHAGEAL DYSFUNCTION

Dysfunction of the esophageal stage of deglutition also must be considered in patients with dysphagia and aspiration. To evaluate the esophageal function the following studies should be obtained: cine-esophageal barium swallow, esophageal manometric measurements, pH testing (because subtle acid reflux is apparent on manometrics), and endoscopy. Extrinsic or intrinsic structural obstruction of the esophagus must be identified. Neuromuscular dysfunction of the esophagus may be described as diffuse esophageal spasm, megaesophagus, lower esophageal achalasia, or hypotensive lower esophageal sphincter with esophageal reflux (Ellis, 1980). By precise manometric measurements in patients with spasm of the esophageal body, functional obstruction can be identified at the point of highest resistance. Surgical intervention by extensive esophageal myotomy of the involved segment is indicated when dysphagia is severe and medical treatment has been unsuccessful. The esophagus is approached through a left thoracotomy incision. As in the cricopharyngeus myotomy, the circular fibers of the esophageal musculature are identified and divided longitudinally over the area of dysfunction.

Megaesophagus resulting from increased resting tension of the lower esophageal sphincter and lower esophageal achalasia are treated effectively by surgical intervention using the modified Heller procedure (Asherson, 1950). A myotomy is performed at the level of the gastroesophageal junction either transthoracically or transabdominally, depending on the necessity for a combined procedure. In cases of megaesophagus where significant dilatation of the esophagus has been demonstrated preoperatively, partial resection of the esophagus is indicated (Negus, 1962; Nicks, 1976). Evaluation of patients following myotomy reveals 18 to 34 percent incidence of gastroesophageal reflux. Complications from esophageal reflux include esophagitis with stricture formation, profound discomfort, and reflex upper esophageal sphincter achalasia (Ellis, 1980; Vantrappen and Hellemans, 1980). The mechanism of increased upper esophageal sphincter tension in esophageal reflux is attributed to chronic irritation of the esophagus followed by a neurogenic reflex tightening of the sphincter (Henderson and Marryatt, 1977). Because of the high incidence of morbidity associated with reflux following a cardiomyotomy, Mansour and co-workers (1976) advocate a combined procedure including a reflux-retarding procedure at the time of myotomy. In addition to being treated for lower esophageal achalasia by myotomy, patients who have primary esophageal reflux from a hypotensive lower esophageal sphincter benefit from an antireflux procedure. Several types are commonly practiced, including the Belsey "Mark IV" transthoracic reconstruction of the cardia, the Nisson fundoplication, and the Hill procedure.

In the medically compromised patient with lower esophageal achalasia, dilatation of the cardia may be an effective alternative. A forceful dilation of the sphincter is necessary using either the Starck dilator, which consists of a balloon of fixed diameter, or the Sippy pneumatic dilator bag (Vantrappen and Hellemans, 1980). Following repeated dilatations, patients experience improvement in dysphagia in 75 percent of cases, with significant reflux occurring only 1 percent of the time (Vantrappen and Hellemans, 1980). The factor limiting the wider use of dilatation techniques is the relatively high (5 percent) incidence of esophageal perforation. Dilatation of the lower esophageal sphincter is effective and should be performed in patients suffering from severe dysphagia who are not candidates for a major operative procedure.

SURGICAL INTERVENTION IN PERSISTENT DYSPHAGIA

A complete myotomy may be ineffective in eliminating the life-threatening problems of dysphagia and aspiration in the most severely debilitated patients. The upper aerodigestive tract fails to perform its role of providing both protected ventilation of the lungs and a passageway for alimentation. Separation of these functions by surgical intervention is required for the patient's survival.

Surgical intervention to provide adequate feedings without associated aspiration include pharyngoesophagostomy, flap esophagostomy, gastrostomy, and jejunostomy (Table 10.2). A nasogastric tube is an effective temporary means to provide adequate nutrition in the debilitated or unconscious patient who has the problem of significant aspiration. Long-term use of the nasogastric tube is limited by discomfort, bleeding, and irritation resulting in increased mucous membrane secretions, regurgitation of feedings, and impairment of pharyngeal swallow (Acquarelli, Fenno, and Ward, 1972).

Esophagostomy

The pharyngoesophagostomy is an effective means of long-term tube feeding and in some patients provides control of secretions in the pharynx that are difficult to manage (Skolnik, Tenta, and Massair, 1966). A fistula is created from the hypopharynx to the skin anterior to the sternocleidomastoid muscle. A Levin tube or similar feeding tube is placed through the fistula tract into the stomach (Figure 10.3). If secretions in the pharynx pose a life-threatening condition because of recurrent aspiration, the fistula tract can be constructed

Table 10.2.   Surgical Routes for Tube Feeding.

Procedure	Advantages	Disadvantages
Esophagostomy	Minimal skin care, tube out between meals, feedings taken upright; reversible as office procedure	Contraindicated in esophageal obstruction, irradiated neck, superior vena cava syndrome
Gastrostomy	Standard procedure; preferable in children	Skin care often troublesome; patient must disrobe for feeding
Jejunostomy	Minimizes gastroesophageal reflux	Increased diarrhea
Pharyngotomy	Local anesthesia, minimal risk	Stoma high in neck, tube changing often difficult

Reprinted by permission of the publisher, from Doby, *American Family Physician,* 1978.

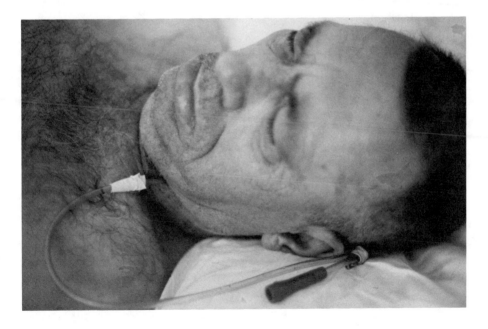

Figure 10.3.   Patient with a cervical esophagostoma in place following a brainstem cerebrovascular accident. Note the marked bilateral facial weakness.

to provide adequate drainage of the hypopharynx to avoid pooling and secondary aspiration. Several modifications of the esophagostomy are now practiced. The skin flap technique (Dobie, Cox, and Larsen, 1979) lines the fistula tract with a skin flap, providing a more permanent fistula and allowing the feeding tube to be removed for short periods of time. Graham and Royster (1967) described a surgical technique that allows placement of a pharyngotomy tube into the pyriform sinus. This procedure, performed under local anesthesia at the bedside, is ideal for the compromised patient who requires urgent placement of a feeding tube and cannot tolerate general anesthesia or abdominal placement.

Advantages of the esophagostoma over the gastrostoma tube are avoidance of an abdominal procedure, use of local anesthesia, the ability to feed the patient in the sitting rather than supine position, and the ability to begin feedings immediately following the procedure. There are several disadvantages of an esophagostomy tube. In addition to local irritation to skin, there is general contraindication in patients with tumor, severe venous congestion in the neck, esophageal obstruction or significant reflux, significant lower respiratory disease and/or dyspnea or frequent cough, and frequent emesis or extensive gastroesophageal reflux.

Gastrostomy

The most common surgical approach for placement of a feeding tube is gastrostomy (Figure 10.4). The popularity of the feeding gastrostomy is best explained by mentioning some of its advantages. The feeding tube is away from the head and neck and therefore can be placed in patients with head and neck or esophageal tumor. A gastrostomy is technically a straightforward procedure that can be done under local anesthesia. Peristomal irritation is less significant than that of the head and neck region.

In patients with significant esophageal reflux, the gastrostomy, pharyngoesophagostomy, and nasogastric feeding tube should be avoided, as they increase the likelihood of postprandial reflux and aspiration. An exception is the new soft, Silastic pediatric feeding tubes that have proved quite valuable in providing total parenteral nutrition.

Jejunostomy

When esophageal reflux and associated aspiration are strongly suspected by history or demonstrated by attempted feeding with a nasogastric tube, a feeding jejunostoma tube is indicated. As with gastrostomy, placement of the jejunostoma tube requires an abdominal procedure, but differs in that a general anesthesia usually is required (Liffman and Randall, 1972). Early selection of the appropriate mode of tube placement in the patient with severe dysphagia is a necessity to prevent starvation and aspiration pneumonia associated with attempted feedings.

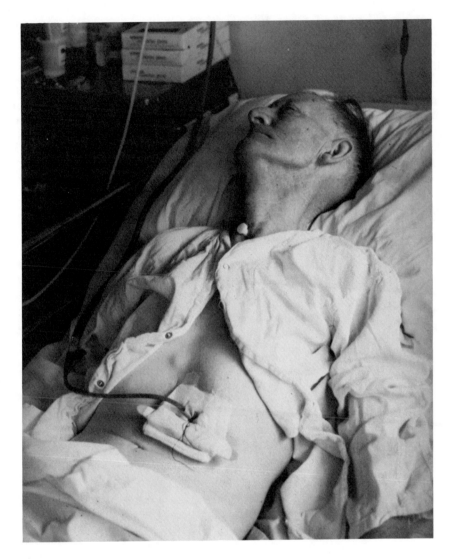

Figure 10.4. Patient with a feeding gastrostoma. Nutrition must be administered with the patient in the recumbent position.

Laryngeal Paralysis

In severe dysfunction of the upper aerodigestive tract, a more immediate problem than establishing a mode for feedings is protection of the airway from life-threatening aspiration. The primary function of the larynx is to act as a sphincter for the airway, preventing the aspiration of secretions and food. To provide normal function, the supraglottic mucous membrane, which is innervated by the internal branch of the superior laryngeal nerve, must respond to the presence of foreign material or secretions by initiating glottic closure. This also is accomplished by stimulation of the trachea. To complete the sphincter-like action, the intrinsic musculature of the larynx that is innervated by the recurrent laryngeal nerve approximates the vocal cords, tightly closing the glottis. Surgical intervention to manage partial or total laryngeal paralysis must be selective based on the degree of paralysis present.

Unilateral low vagal paralysis below the level of the nodose ganglion results initially in paramedian-positioned vocal cords, producing hoarseness and minimal aspiration (Figure 10.5). In the late stage of paralysis the vocal cords move to the abducted position as the ipsilateral muscles slowly atrophy (Sasaki, 1980). In this position the patient may experience mild aspiration and marked hoarseness. By injecting Teflon into the paralyzed cord, (Rontal

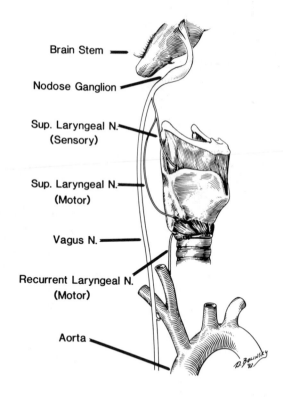

Brain Stem

Nodose Ganglion

Sup. Laryngeal N.
(Sensory)

Sup. Laryngeal N.
(Motor)

Vagus N.

Recurrent Laryngeal N.
(Motor)

Aorta

Figure 10.5. Branches of the vagus (superior and recurrent laryngeal nerves) that innervate the sensory and motor aspects of the larynx. Loss of sensory and motor innervation above and below the level of the nodose ganglion produces different pathology.
Drawing by David Bolinsky.

et al., 1976) partial closure of the glottic space usually results in improved voice and decreased aspiration.

Teflon Injection

Using the Arnold-Breuning syringe, approximately 0.25 cc of Teflon paste is injected into the paralyzed vocal cord at two points: one at the middle third of the cord and one above the vocal process of the arytenoid (Figure 10.6). The procedure is performed under local anesthesia with visualization of the vocal cords being obtained by suspension laryngoscopy. By moving the paralyzed cord to the median position, voice quality is markedly improved and aspiration may be decreased. Prior to injecting Teflon, the surgeon may elect to inject absorbable gelatin sponge (Gelfoam) into the paralyzed vocal cord to anticipate the more permanent effects of Teflon. Gelfoam injections usually are made with patients who are expected to have return of function or when there is a question as to the efficacy of Teflon. We prefer to use Teflon in patients with carcinoma and generalized neurologic deficits because this is a quick, easy procedure, and it does not seem prudent to do any more than one procedure on patients in this group due to the increased morbidity rate.

Nerve-to-Muscle Pedicle

In bilateral low vagal paralysis, deglutition is rarely impaired and aspiration is a minimal problem as the vocal cords tend to be in the median position.

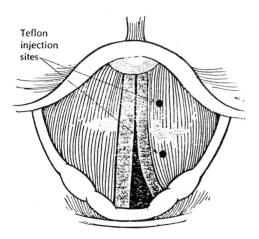

Teflon injection sites

Figure 10.6. Superior view of the vocal cords illustrating the Teflon injection sites on the paralyzed vocal cord. Reprinted by permission of the publisher, from Doby, *American Family Physician*, 1978.

Initial therapy involves providing an adequate airway and protecting against aspiration by the placement of a cuffed tracheostoma tube. Improved respiration may be accomplished by fixed lateralization of one of the paralyzed cords. By permanently widening the glottic space for increased respiration, aspiration will increase and may pose a difficult management problem. An alternative surgical approach that is becoming more popular is the use of a nerve-to-muscle pedicle transferred from the omohyoid muscle to the paralyzed posterior cricoarytenoid (Tucker, 1976). Inspiratory activity of the omohyoideus mediated by the ansa hypoglossi results in phasic vocal cord abduction, which may be adequate to allow increased ventilation and at the same time protect the airway against aspiration.

Tympanic Neurectomy

High unilateral vagus paralysis above the nodose ganglion results in vocal cord and pharyngeal paralysis that produces significant dysphagia and aspiration of stagnated material retained in the hypopharynx (see Figure 10.5). Surgical intervention in these cases requires a combination of procedures to facilitate deglutition and protect the airway from aspiration.

Initially, a cuffed tracheostoma tube is placed, followed by the insertion of a feeding tube, Teflon injection of the paralyzed vocal cord, and cricopharyngeal myotomy (Glenn et al., 1980). If persistent aspiration of secretions in the pharynx continues, bilateral chorda tympani and tympanic nerve sections may be performed by a transtympanic approach under local anesthesia (Mills, 1975; Townsend, Morimoto, and Kralemann, 1973). By sectioning the chorda tympani and tympanic nerve, the parasympathetic innervation of the submandibular and parotid glands is interrupted, markedly decreasing the oral secretions (Figure 10.7). These nerve sections often are effective in controlling secretions, but approximately 30 percent of patients have a recurrence of symptoms in the first six months following operation.

Laryngeal Closure

In high bilateral vagal nerve paralysis, immediate airway control is required to maintain life. As soon as is practical, a cuffed tracheostoma tube and a feeding tube, usually gastrostoma, are placed. In the past, this condition and cases where the ninth, tenth, eleventh, and twelfth cranial nerves are involved required laryngectomy to prevent recurrent aspiration, pneumonia, and death. There are now alternative procedures including diversion of the larynx (Lindeman, 1975), an epiglottic flap (sewing the epiglottis over the false cords into the arytenoids) (Habal and Murray, 1972), and laryngeal closure (Sasaki et al., 1980). The most practical and effective approach is the laryngeal closure described by Montgomery (1975) and modified by Sasaki (1980).

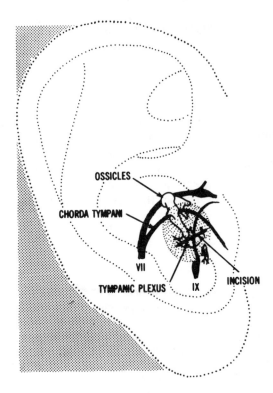

OSSICLES

CHORDA TYMPANI

VII

TYMPANIC PLEXUS   IX   INCISION

Figure 10.7. Diagram of the parasympathetic nerve supply to the major salivary glands
and their accessibility within the middle
ear. Tympanic neurectomy is performed
within the tympanic plexus. Reprinted by
permission of the publisher, from DeLisa et
al., *American Family Physician,* 1979.

Both close the larynx and are reversible if there is significant neurologic
improvement.

Following placement of a permanent tracheostoma, a horizontal skin
incision over the cricoid is made to approach the larynx. The larynx is entered
by a vertical midline thyrotomy. Mucous membrane between the free edges
of the vocal and vestibular folds is resected. The glottis is then closed beginning superiorly by approximating the denuded edges of the vestibular
folds. A superior-based sternohyoid muscle pedicle is then passed through
the thyroid notch and sutured to the interarytenoideus muscle at the posterior
commissure. The vocal folds are then approximated, followed by closure of
the thyrotomy and the skin incision. By the placement of the sternohyoid
muscle pedicle, the dead space between the vocal and vestibular folds is
eliminated and the larynx is closed in three layers. Laryngeal closure effec-

tively protects the respiratory tract from aspiration while allowing the upper aerodigestive tract to be used for alimentation.

SUMMARY

The management of deglutition disorders may be significantly aided by surgical intervention. The goals of specific surgical procedures are to protect the airway from aspiration, to facilitate deglutition, or to provide an alternative mode of alimentation. Appropriate surgical intervention is determined by the patient's symptoms and degree of debilitation. By early awareness of the need for surgical intervention, the morbidity and mortality of deglutition disorders may be decreased.

REFERENCES

Acquarelli MJ, Fenno G, Ward PH. Cervical esophagostomy (an improved technique for alimentation of the debilitated patient). Arch Otolaryngol 1972;96:453–56.

Asherson N. Achalasia of the cricopharyngeal sphincter: record of cases, with profile pharyngograms. J Laryngol Otol 1950;64:747–58.

Black RJ. Cricopharyngeal myotomy. J Otolaryngol 1981;10:145–48.

Blakley WR, Garety EJ, Smith DE. Section of the cricopharyngeus muscle for dysphagia. Arch Surg 1968;96:745–60.

Calcaterra JC, Kadell BM, Ward PH. Dysphagia secondary to cricopharyngeal muscle dysfunction. Arch Otolaryngol 1975;101:726–29.

Chodosh PL. Cricopharyngeal myotomy in the treatment of dysphagia. Laryngoscope 1975;85:1862–73.

DeLisa JA, Mikulic MA, Miller RM, Melnick RR. Amyotrophic lateral sclerosis: comprehensive management. Am Fam Physician 1979;19:137–42.

Dobie RA, Cox KW, Larsen GL. Skin flap esophagostomy: a new procedure. Arch Otolaryngol 1979;105:200–2.

Doby R. Rehabilitation of swallowing disorders. Am Fam Physician 1978;17:84–95.

Dohlman G, Mattson O. The endoscopic operation of hypopharyngeal diverticula: a roentgenocinematographic study. Arch Otolaryngol 1960;71;744–52.

Ellis FH. Upper esophageal sphincter in health and disease. Surg Clin North Am 1971;51:553–65.

Ellis FH. Surgical management of esophageal motility disturbances. Am J Surg 1980;139:752–59.

Ellis FH Jr, Schlegel JF, Lynch VP, Payne WS. Cricopharyngeal myotomy for pharyngo-esophageal diverticulum. Ann Surg 1969;170:340–49.

English GM. Otolaryngology. New York: Harper & Row, 1980.

Glenn WWL, Hoak B, Sasaki C, Kirchner JA. Characteristics and surgical management of respiratory complications accompanying pathologic lesions of the brainstem. Ann Surg 1980;191:655–63.

Graham W, Royster HP. Simplified cervical esophagostomy for long-term extraoral feeding. Surg Gynecol Obstet 1967;125:127–28.

Habal MB, Murray JE. Surgical treatment of life endangering chronic aspiration pneumonia. Plast Reconstr Surg 1972;49:305–11.

Henderson RD, Marryatt G. Cricopharyngeal myotomy as a method of treating cricopharyngeal dysphagia secondary to gastro-esophageal reflux. J Thorac Cardiovasc Surg 1977;74:721–25.

Hollinshead WH. Anatomy for surgeons. New York: Harper & Row, 1968.

Kirchner JA. The motor activity of the cricopharyngeus muscle. Laryngoscope 1958;68:1119–59.

Lebo CP, Kwei SU, Norris PH. Cricopharyngeal myotomy in amyotrophic lateral sclerosis. Laryngoscope 1976;86:862–68.

Liffmann KE, Randall HT. A modified technique for creating a jejunostomy. Surg Gynecol Obstet 1972;134:663–64.

Lindeman RC. Overting the paralyzed larynx: a reversible procedure for intractable aspiration. Laryngoscope 1975;85:157–80.

Lund WS. The cricopharyngeal sphincter: its relationship to the relief of pharyngeal paralysis and the surgical treatment of early pharyngeal pouch. J Laryngol 1968;82:353–67.

Mansour KA, Symbas P, Ellis J, Matache C. A combined surgical approach in the management of achalasia of the esophagus. Ann Surg 1976;42:192–95.

Mills CP. Cricopharyngeal sphincterotomy and bilateral division of the chorda tympani in bulbar palsy. Proc R Soc Med 1975;68:644–46.

Montgomery WW. Surgery to prevent aspiration. Arch Otolaryngol 1975;101:679–82.

Negus VE. Comparative anatomy and physiology of the larynx. New York: Hafner, 1962.

Nicks GR. Webs, dysrhythmias and diverticula of the esophagus. NZ Med J 1976;84:179–83.

Orringer MB. Extended cervical esophagomyotomy for cricopharyngeal dysfunction. J Thorac Cardiovasc Surg 1980;30:669–78.

Rontal E, Rontal M, Morse G, et al. Vocal cord injection in the treatment of acute and chronic aspiration. Laryngoscope 1976;86:625–34.

Sasaki CT. Paralysis of the larynx and pharynx. Surg Clin North Am 1980;60:1079–92.

Sasaki CT, Milmoe G, Yanagisawa E, Berry K, Kirchner JA. Surgical closure of the larynx for intractable aspiration. Arch Otolaryngol 1980;106:422–23.

Skolnik EM, Tenta LT, Massair FS. Pharyngo-esophagostomy. Arch Otolaryngol 1966;84:534–37.

Thawley SE, Ogura JH. Cricopharyngeal myotomy. Laryngoscope 1978;88:872–74.

Townsend G, Morimoto AM, Kralemann H. Management of sialorrhea by trans-tympanic neurectomy. Mayo Clin Proc 1973;48:776–79.

Tucker HM. Human laryngeal reinnervation. Laryngoscope 1976;86:769–79.

Vantrappen G, Hellemans J. Treatment of achalasia and related motor disorders. Gastroenterology 1980;79:144–54.

Weaver AW, Fleming SM. Partial laryngectomy: analysis of associated swallowing disorders. Am J Surg 1978;136:486–89.

Zuckerbraum L, Bahma MS. Cricopharyngeus myotomy as the only treatment for Zenker's diverticulum. Ann Otol 1979;88:798–803.

CHAPTER 11

Establishing a Swallowing Program

Michael E. Groher and Ina Elfant Asher

It may seem somewhat ironic that this book ends with a discussion devoted to beginning a swallowing program. The preceding chapters help to provide the clinician with the basic theoretical and technical knowledge needed to evaluate and treat swallowing disorders. A thorough and working understanding of the issues and topics discussed is the first step in developing a program. It is necessary to become familiar with the literature and professional staff involved, and with the evaluation and treatment procedures recommended. All can serve as important resources when problems and questions arise.

Putting this knowledge into place in a clinical setting may be the greatest challenge of all. This chapter focuses directly on organizing and developing a dysphagia program. Clinicians who have had direct experience in managing swallowing disorders on a regular basis would agree that there are certain key organizational steps that must be taken. By accepting the fact that good dysphagia programs do not evolve overnight we can adjust to the potential psychologic disappointments that may be frequent in the initial stages. Our program took three full years before it became a viable and recognized part of the hospital's life. Others have taken longer.

ESTABLISHING GOALS

There are many kinds of programs that can be established. Each of the contributors to this book has had a different experience, whether in a hospital-wide, multidisciplinary dysphagia clinic, or as a single therapist incorporating the techniques into a personal schedule of rehabilitation treatment. The size and type of patient population, attitudes of the staff toward rehabilitation, available personnel, the real opportunity for program development, and most important, individual interest in dysphagia are essential considerations in defining a program suitable to a particular setting. The type of program ultimately established will depend on the goals defined.

Three goals should be universal to all dysphagia programs: (1) identification of the patient who may be at risk for aspiration (2) prevention of aspiration, and (3) prevention of malnutrition. The minimal requirement of the staff to achieve these goals is careful evaluation and re-evaluation of the patient to determine the extent to which oral foods are tolerated. It can be argued that the additional goal of improvement of swallowing behavior be included whenever possible.

Ideally, the patient should achieve a nutritionally complete oral diet. If this is not possible, nonoral supplements or total feedings should be recommended. We believe that the rudiments of a successful dysphagia program can be established based on evaluation and careful monitoring to achieve the first three goals. It is our preference, however, to attempt the active intervention described in the treatment chapters where potential for improvement has not been ruled out.

Depending upon the capabilities of the staff and the extent to which the dysphagia program is incorporated into general rehabilitation, other goals may be expressed, for example, increasing the patient's independence in eating (or in self-administration of tube feedings) and assisting the family to care for the patient's special nutritional needs at home.

ASSEMBLING A TEAM

The contributors to this book are representatives of diverse fields of health care management, all with a common interest in swallowing disorders. Those in other disciplines such as gastroenterology, radiology, social service, surgery, respiratory therapy, and physical therapy also have an interest. Dysphagia management will be maximized if each participate, either directly and on a daily basis or by periodic consultations. If possible, an individual or individuals from each service can be identified who have a particular interest in dysphagia and who can serve as direct resource persons for consultations or in-service training. For a section head or supervisor to give tacit approval for the department as a whole to participate is not as useful as specifically designating an individual to be an active representative.

The continuity of care and specialization of knowledge needed to manage dysphagic patients is facilitated if one individual assumes direct responsibility and it is clear to the rest of the team who that individual is. This person will be the most visible member and therefore the one to whom consultations will be directed. The team leader probably will be the prime participator in dysphagia management on a daily basis. Responsibilities usually include accepting consultations, completing the evaluation with appropriate recommendations, coordinating the necessary rehabilitation or further diagnostic tests, and providing some direct feeding training. It is our feeling that the team leader will eventually have to devote 35 to 45 percent of total working hours to dysphagia management if employed in a hospital or rehabilitation center setting.

The role played by each member of the dysphagia management team may differ from clinic to clinic; however, most contributions are established as part of traditional roles. A specialized interest or demonstrated expertise in dysphagia management may lead to some overlapping of responsibilities. This should not be viewed by other team members as encroachment, but rather as the best way to provide swallowing rehabilitation for patients. Some dysphagia rehabilitation programs have failed to sustain themselves because of the failure of team members to define and accept their roles. The following may help to serve as useful guidelines.

Nursing Staff

The nurses, through physician orders, have the direct responsibility of monitoring the patient's medical and nutritional status. In many institutions, they coordinate dysphagia consultations and as such serve as a dysphagia team leader. Overall responsibilities usually include administration and care of nonoral feeding including hyperalimentation and tube feedings, recording oral and nonoral intake (particularly of fluids), care and suctioning of tracheostoma tubes, maintaining good oral hygiene, and assigning nursing staff or volunteers to assist with feeding at mealtimes. Nurses should be responsible, in part, for reporting successes and failures during oral feedings. These impressions are recorded in the progress notes.

Occupational Therapist

Concern for manual feeding skills has been a traditional part of an occupational therapist's involvement in improving the patient's daily living skills. Experience in training patients with motor weakness or loss of function to adapt to new feeding techniques has often led the occupational therapist to coordinate dysphagic rehabilitation. This therapist is a specialist in suggesting which types of adaptive equipment would be best suited for the patient's needs and in providing specific technical assistance at mealtimes in addition to being well trained in general physical rehabilitation techniques. In conjunction with the physical therapist, the occupational therapist may provide preliminary therapy to reduce muscle spasticity, improve muscle strength and coordination, and prevent primitive reflex patterns from interfering with swallowing.

Dietitian

The dietitian monitors the patient's overall nutritional status, ensuring that the patient's intake of fluids and nutrients meets the requirements as appropriate to the medical condition. The dietitian coordinates special diet orders with the kitchen, assists in obtaining a dysphagia evaluation tray, takes a dietary history when possible, and makes specific recommendations relating to food textures and nutritional values. If the patient is receiving tube feedings, the dietitian can make recommendations about the type, adequacy, and regulation of the feedings.

The dietitian is the most important resource when treatment involves provision of specialized nutritional and food technological requirements. An example might be to combine foods that provide high-caloric or low-salt content with gelatin to facilitate swallowing, together with some special spices to appeal to the patient's taste. This person who serves as the liaison between the team and the kitchen may find it useful to develop a dysphagia diet order sheet to be used by the team (Figure 11.1).

Speech Pathologist

Many patients with swallowing difficulty also have accompanying disorders of speech production. It follows that the speech pathologist would become directly involved with both the diagnosis and management of dysphagic patients. Many times the patient's swallowing disorder must be managed before speech rehabilitation can begin. The speech pathologist is expert in muscle reeducation of the oral and laryngeal structures. In many institutions the speech pathologist is the team leader.

Neurologist

The neurologist is one of the primary diagnosticians on the swallowing management team. It is this person's responsibility to help differentiate neurologic from mechanical and psychogenic swallowing disorders. The neurologist combines the results of physical examination with those of radiography, electromyography, electroneurography, and muscle and nerve biopsy to arrive at an etiologic diagnosis. Recommendations for special techniques may be combined with prescribing medications that assist in swallowing management by modification of the neurologic disease.

Otolaryngologist

The otolaryngologist has a special interest in the differential diagnosis of mechanical swallowing disorders. Usually he is the most familiar with the sensory and motor abnormalities of the pharynx and larynx. This includes surgical management of the majority of head and neck cancers and post-

Directions:
1. Circle desired foods.
2. 24-hour notice is required for food preparation.
3. Notify appropriate staff dietitian regarding revisions.
4. Only signed and dated order sheets will be accepted.
5. Send to dietary department.

SWALLOWING TRAINING	CHEWING TRAINING

1. Stiff jelled:
   Pureed meat
   Pureed vegetables
   Fruit
2. Standard jelled:
   Jello
   Custard
   Pudding
3. Purees:
   Meats
   Mashed potato
   Vegetables
   Squash
   Fruits
   Plain or vanilla yogurt
   Poached egg
   Oatmeal
   Cream of Wheat
   Applesauce
4. Thick liquids:
   Ice cream
   Sherbet
   High-protein frappes
   Thickened cream soups
   Thinned pureed fruits
   High-protein eggnog
   Carnation Instant Breakfast
   Thinned Cream of Wheat
5. Clear liquids:
   (All clear liquids including gelatin)
	6. Dysphagia—mechanical soft:
	   Ground meat
	   Flaked fish
	   Tuna, egg, or chicken salad
	   Toast
	   Cottage cheese
	   Soft canned fruit
	   Poached egg
	   Scrambled egg
	   Omelette, plain
	   Macaroni and cheese
	   Peanut butter
	7. Chunk consistency*:
	   Diced meats
	   Chopped vegetables
	   Soft diced fruits
	   Crackers
	   Cookies (Arrowroot)
	
	*Additional food items from earlier swallowing training (e.g., juice or cereal) may be added to provide nutrient needs and variety.

Requested by:_____ Date:_____

Figure 11.1. Swallowing training diet sheet.

surgical swallowing disorders and subsequent nutritional status. The otolaryngologist may perform specialized surgical procedures such as myotomy or esophagostomy to manage persistent dysphagia.

Gastroenterologist

The gastroenterologist serves as a diagnostician and surgical consultant for patients with suspected dysphagia related to the esophagus and/or gastrointestinal tract. While usually not directly involved in daily dysphagia management, an interested gastroenterologist can be an important member of the swallowing management team.

Respiratory Therapist

The respiratory therapist is not usually directly involved on the dysphagia team, but does provide valuable information relating to patients with respiratory disorders and tracheostoma tubes. This includes monitoring pulmonary toilet and assisting the physician by making recommendations for removal of the tracheostoma tube. Often this therapist will provide expert consultation on the choice of tracheostoma tube and how it should be used during feedings.

Attending Physician

Although each patient's attending or primary physician is not necessarily a member of the dysphagia team, all communications must include this person. The physician as coordinator of the patient's total medical and surgical management must order the original consultation to the dysphagia team or medical specialist. Within each facility, it is imperative for orders to be written clearly. The dysphagia evaluation should be prescribed specifically. If the patient is a candidate for oral intake, the orders should reflect the physician's concurrence because of the potential risks of aspiration and subsequent illness. Any changes in dietary management should also be accompanied by written orders. The question of liability is often the first issue to be raised when a dysphagia program is introduced in a new setting. The primary care physician must be in agreement with each step involved in the patient's dysphagia management.

TIME ASSESSMENT

The amount of time needed to serve as team leader may appear excessive, especially for the individual who is already fully involved in specialized patient care. The team leader should first try to free this amount of time through direct reassignment of responsibilities within the hospital or clinic. If this is not possible, the dysphagia team may need to consider the recruitment and training of nursing assistants or hospital volunteers.

The major activity in a dysphagia rehabilitation program is feeding patients at mealtimes. Although this should be overseen by the team leader, feeding training sessions may be carried out by assigned (trained) nursing or therapy personnel. Volunteers should be so assigned only after a patient has demonstrated repeated success at swallowing and requires no more than standby assistance. The drain in terms of time on staff who are involved in training volunteers or directly involved in feeding at mealtimes may be exorbitant. Weekends and holidays are the most difficult times for program coordination and implementation. Therefore, the need arises to develop a dependable corps of trained volunteers or family members who can be instructed to follow a prescribed feeding program without direct assistance.

Team members also must make some personal commitments to changes in their work schedules. The hours of eight to four and nine to five with an hour off for lunch are incompatible with care of dysphagia patients. Most in-patient settings serve meals at 7 A.M., noon, and 5 P.M. Therefore if one is to assist in feeding, consideration must be given to rearrangement of working hours.

IDENTIFYING THE POPULATION

A dysphagia team may wish to limit the scope of its initial efforts to a small segment or service of the hospital population; for example, rehabilitation, neurology, and otolaryngology. The team might decide to run a demonstration diagnostic and treatment dysphagia program on one of these services in an effort to evaluate the efficacy of beginning such a program and to eliminate some of the problems that can arise as it is established.

As the program develops, the need for diagnostic and swallowing treatment services will become apparent. One consultation a week will quickly turn into five and perhaps ten, as word of its existence spreads. Based on data gathered from charge nurses in an 800-bed acute care hospital, approximately 6 percent (48 patients) had an identifiable swallowing disorder at some time during their stay (Groher, 1980). Approximately half of these patients will actually require diagnostic or swallowing treatment services. The remaining 3 percent have either persistent swallowing disorders that have been managed previously or cannot benefit from rehabilitation due to the severity of their disease. It has been our experience that dysphagia programs in the initial stages will usually treat 12 to 15 patients per week.

Growth of the program depends upon available staff time and efficient coordination of team effort. Team members who can spend only a limited amount of time per day with dysphagic patients normally will limit their efforts to those who can benefit the most. The same principle holds true for those very active programs that attempt to provide services to more patients than their resources can support.

Some centers have found it necessary to provide outpatient clinics for patients who continue to have episodes of dysphagia following hospital discharge, and for those who do not need hospitalization but who complain specifically of swallowing difficulty. Such clinics require additional space and staff time, both of which must be carefully budgeted. The majority of patients who are candidates for swallowing rehabilitation do recover during their hospital course (Groher, 1980), minimizing the need for additional outpatient visits. Clinics are usually formed only after the dysphagia program has become well recognized both in the hospital and in the immediate community.

OUTLINING THE PROGRAM AND PROCEDURES

At this point it should be possible to outline the structure of the dysphagia program in terms of who will participate, how much they will participate, where they will participate, and finally, the rationale for beginning such an effort. This information is usually passed through the hospital's appropriate chain of command for final approval. A statement of procedures is a useful attachment to the program outline. The following are questions for consideration:

1. How will dysphagic patients be identified?
2. To whom will consultations and follow-up orders be directed?
3. What is the process for constructing and ordering a swallowing evaluation diet?
4. Will the need to have dysphagic patients eat smaller portions more times per day require procedural changes between the dietary service and the kitchen?
5. Who will be responsible for monitoring the results of dysphagia rehabilitation?
6. How are the results to be documented?
7. What medical precautions must be taken when dysphagia therapy is initiated?

The final point requires some elaboration. As pointed out in Chapter 4, one can minimize risks of aspiration after introducing food orally by completing a thorough evaluation of the patient's neuromuscular and cortical potentials before beginning. Patients can and do aspirate during trial periods of swallowing rehabilitation, and the dysphagia team must delineate the types of precautions to be taken. This includes knowledge of suctioning and emergency medical procedures and, of course, clearance from the attending physician. Some centers begin by having the attending physician or registered nurse present during all first-time attempts at oral feeding; as the feeder becomes more experienced, this support may not be as necessary. The therapist who provides feeding training should receive special clinical privileges from the hospital's chief of staff before independent first-time feedings begin.

Finally, a pilot study might be initiated at this stage with permission from the appropriate medical or research committee. When the program has been outlined and the dysphagia team has become familiar with the procedures, such a study may facilitate final acceptance of the program. A small sample of patients should be drawn from those who are identified as being most in need of the team's services. Physicians who support the program may be enlisted to refer candidates from among their patients. For example, a neurologist may refer a patient who has recently had a cerebrovascular accident. By carefully documenting evaluation and treatment results, the team will be able to make a preliminary assessment of the success of the program. Dysphagia management procedures then can be finalized.

INITIATING THE PROGRAM

After final approval has been given, announcements should be sent to each service director and ward physician briefly describing the program's intent and consultation procedures.

At this point, training should begin, focusing on the types of services the team will offer and their importance to the patient's medical recovery. Training should be offered first to staff physicians and nurses. It is best accomplished if the physician and nursing members of the dysphagia team teach their peers; however, to enhance collaboration and improve the visibility of the program, the team leader should be included in all educational sessions. Members from the allied health sector (dietetics, speech pathology, rehabilitation) can provide training to their own peers and can assist in training volunteers to serve as feeders. Publicity should be ongoing to alert nonrelated hospital staff and consumers that such a specialized program exists. This may be especially important in active medical centers with constant changes of house staff assignments. Grand rounds presentations and hospital newsletter articles can communicate achievements as well as assist in gaining wider acceptance of the program.

Volunteer training should focus on the basics of the swallowing act and the importance of strictly adhering to the prescription for feeding designed by the rehabilitation team. Such prescriptions should be clearly posted at bedside with a copy in the nursing files to facilitate communication among day, evening, and night shifts. Each prescription should be clearly signed and provide an appropriate telephone or call number of a person to contact for additional assistance. An example of such a prescription is as follows:

1. Make sure patient is sitting upright during and one-half hour after eating.
2. Pull curtains around bed to minimize distractions.
3. Let the patient feed himself making sure he takes one bite and swallows before taking another. He will require reminders to do so.
4. Do not talk with the patient while he is eating as this serves as a distraction and interferes with swallowing.
   For more information call: R. Y., Ex. 212

Beeper: 303

When appropriate, the prescription should also include the types of foods and liquids that are and are not permitted. This helps to eliminate confusion that may result from a patient receiving the wrong food tray. These prescriptions greatly facilitate the passing of information from shift to shift and from volunteer to volunteer, as most volunteers do not come each day, nor do they always feed the same patients.

The team leader should monitor any changes needed in diets and/or procedures for feeding. Ideally, one member from the dysphagia team makes rounds with the ward physicians to report progress in dysphagia rehabilitation and to keep informed of changes in the patient's medical status that may preclude oral feeding or dictate different nutritional requirements. The importance of passing clear and relevant information from the team leader to the nursing staff and volunteers cannot be underestimated. Dysphagia rehabilitation efforts can change from day to day, and unless requests and orders are easily translated and implemented, they can be hampered and lead to undue frustration.

MAINTAINING RECORDS

Daily notes are generally kept by physicians and therapists, while nurses record progress notes for each shift. The team leader should ensure that progress is addressed at least once a day or as often as each meal. An immediate notation should be made on any occurrence or suspicion of significant aspiration, including which staff member was notified and the action taken. Immediate notation should also be made after diet changes, either to add a newly tolerated food or to delete an item that is not well tolerated. A change in the patient's alertness, physical appearance, metabolism, or mental status, as well as new evaluative findings such as the return or absence of swallowing reflexes should be reported as soon as they are observed.

Routine daily notes should review the gains and/or losses achieved by dysphagia rehabilitation. They should indicate both the training techniques employed and the success or failure of the prescribed diet. The nursing staff and dietitian are usually responsible for recording fluid intake and output. In addition, a daily record of food intake can be charted, identifying the exact quantity of each item actually consumed as closely as can be estimated. Allowance should be made for spillage or drooling, as this may significantly alter estimates made from leftovers on the tray (Figure 11.2).

Close examination of these charts often shows patterns of food intake that might otherwise have gone unnoticed. For instance, it may become clear that a patient seems to swallow best when macaroni rather than ground meat is on the menu. Another patient may swallow better at the noon meal, related to the level of alertness at that particular time, or to the diet or therapist.

Patient's name: _____
Date: _____
Recorder: _____

Breakfast	Lunch	Dinner	Snacks
10 cc tomato juice	60 cc buttered noodles	30 cc ground beef	60 cc eggnog
1 poached egg	60 cc applesauce	60 cc mashed potato	120 cc Jello
60 cc oatmeal	30 cc eggnog	60 cc thickened chowder	
½ pat butter		½ pear (canned)	
30 cc milk			

Figure 11.2. Food consumption chart.

This specific information can prove useful for supporting changes in diet or modifications of training techniques.

Charting food consumption will give a good picture of the patient's progress in eating as well as of daily nutritional intake in the absence of a calorie count. In the event a calorie count is ordered, the dietitian keeps a careful record of the daily calorie intake, usually done over a period of several days (see Chapter 8).

MEASURING RESULTS

If a pilot study is completed before the program begins, a follow-up study should be done to measure the effectiveness of the program in progress. It is essential to determine the program's success in achieving its objectives, such as reducing the incidence of aspiration pneumonias, reducing dependence on tube feedings (measured by days of use or incidence), shortening total dysphagia recovery time, and promoting a normal oral diet (measured by the diet achieved at the conclusion of the program or at discharge).

The dysphagia team must keep careful records on each patient who is referred for evaluation. Maintaining separate files can facilitate data collection for future use. Data should be organized so that they specifically describe the patient population, including age, cause of dysphagia, and significant contributing medical history. Evaluation techniques and results should be coded for each patient. These basic data eventually can be compared with the goals that were originally set. They can also serve as a program evaluation tool or as the basis for scientific investigation.

The study might seek to evaluate treatment techniques, such as the effects manipulation of diet might bring versus only cognitive training without diet manipulation. Unfortunately, some experimental designs of this nature involve depriving a control group of selected intervention. One way to avoid this ethical dilemma is to use the chart audit procedure now routinely performed in many institutions. By establishing outcome criteria for the chart review, a sample can be selected and charts collected from a specific, predetermined time period. A matched group of charts then can be drawn for comparison from a previous time period (prior to initiation of the program, but recent enough to ensure similar medical management). This step is not essential to the chart audit, as the first sample is intended to be measured only against its own criteria. Even if chart audit fails, it provides a valuable tool for identifying and correcting problems that surface during the review. A subsequent reaudit should succeed if the program is, in fact, effective.

Finally, administrators and colleagues must be informed of both the positive and negative results of the studies, as they can be important for keeping the program visible and viable.

SUMMARY

Dysphagia rehabilitation is still in its infancy. The scientific base for understanding the mechanisms involved in the act of swallowing is just emerging. Management of the disordered system is still very much a clinical art unsupported by a scientific data base on large numbers of patients with different conditions and receiving various combinations of treatment modalities. The challenge now is to gather this information so that dysphagia rehabilitation can move ahead on firmer ground in the next decade.

REFERENCE

Groher M. Establishing a need for a dysphagia program. New York: Health Systems Review Organization Review, Veterans Administration Medical Center, 1980.

INDEX